The Intermittent Fasting Guide for Women Over 60

Unlock Vitality, Boost Longevity, and Embrace
Weight Loss for Your Best Years Yet

Amanda Wells

Copyright © 2025 by Amanda Wells

All rights reserved.

No portion of this book may be reproduced in any form without written permission from the publisher or author, except as permitted by U.S. copyright law.

This publication is designed to provide accurate and authoritative information in regard to the subject matter covered. It is sold with the understanding that neither the author nor the publisher is engaged in rendering legal, investment, accounting or other professional services. While the publisher and author have used their best efforts in preparing this book, they make no representations or warranties with respect to the accuracy or completeness of the contents of this book and specifically disclaim any implied warranties of merchantability or fitness for a particular purpose. No warranty may be created or extended by sales representatives or written sales materials. The advice and strategies contained herein may not be suitable for your situation. You should consult with a professional when appropriate. Neither the publisher nor the author shall be liable for any loss of profit or any other commercial damages, including but not limited to special, incidental, consequential, personal, or other damages.

Book Cover by Amanda Wells

Contents

Disclaimer	1
Introduction	3
Welcome to a New Era of Wellness	
The Journey to Holistic Wellness	
1. Understanding Intermittent Fasting	15
What Is Intermittent Fasting?	
How Fasting Works	
Types of Intermittent Fasting	
2. Why Intermittent Fasting Is Ideal for Women Over 60	33
The Evolving Body	
The Long-Term Health Benefits of Fasting	
Challenges and How to Overcome Them	
3. Getting Started with Intermittent Fasting	49
Preparing Mentally and Physically	
How to Personalize Fasting	
Guidelines for Getting Started	
4. Smart Nutrition During Fasting	63
What to Eat When Not Fasting	
Foods That Enhance Fasting	

    What to Avoid

5. Fasting and an Active Lifestyle   81
    The Importance of Physical Activity
    Managing Stress and Sleep
    Creating a Daily Rhythm

6. Testimonials and Inspiration   97
    Success Stories
    Common Mistakes to Avoid

7. Solutions for Specific Situations   105
    Fasting and Health Issues
    Travel and Social Life
    Adjustments for a Flexible Lifestyle

8. Simple Recipes to Support Fasting   117
    Quick and Easy Meals
    Drinks for Fasting

9. Frequently Asked Questions   139
    Answers to the Most Common Concerns
    Debunking Fasting Myths

10. Maintaining Results Over Time   149
    Turning Fasting Into a Habit
    Monitoring Progress
    A Future of Wellness

Conclusion   163
    Celebrating Yourself

Appendices 171
    1. 30-Day Fasting Plan
    3. Glossary of Terms

Bonus Chapter: Your Exclusive Fasting Tools 179

Acknowledgments 181

Disclaimer

This book is intended as an informational and educational guide on **Intermittent Fasting**. It is not a substitute for professional medical advice, diagnosis, or treatment. Before making any changes to your diet, lifestyle, or health routines, it is strongly recommended that you consult with a qualified healthcare professional to assess any potential contraindications or personal sensitivities.

The author is not responsible for any issues, health complications, or consequences that may arise from the interpretation or application of the information presented in this book based on personal decisions. Each individual's health needs are unique, and professional guidance should always be sought before implementing any dietary or lifestyle changes.

Introduction

Welcome to a New Era of Wellness

The History of Intermittent Fasting

Intermittent fasting may seem like a modern wellness trend, but its roots stretch deep into human history. For thousands of years, fasting has been an integral part of human life: not by choice, but by necessity. Before the advent of agriculture and food abundance, early humans often experienced natural periods of fasting as they searched for sustenance. These periods of fasting weren't just survival mechanisms; they also allowed the body to repair itself, conserve energy, and function optimally under challenging conditions.

As civilizations evolved, fasting took on a more structured and intentional role. Across cultures and religions, fasting was practiced not only as a means of survival but also as a tool for spiritual growth and physical health. From the ancient Greeks to the great Eastern traditions, fasting was seen as a way to purify the body and mind. Hippocrates, often called the "Father of Medicine," advocated fasting as a healing method, famously stating, "To eat when you are sick is to feed your illness."

Religious traditions have also preserved the practice of fasting throughout history. For example:

- In Christianity, Lent includes fasting to foster spiritual discipline.
- Islam's holy month of Ramadan involves daily fasting from dawn to sunset as an act of devotion.
- Hinduism and Buddhism also promote fasting as a way to achieve mental clarity and spiritual enlightenment.

In modern times, fasting has moved beyond its historical and spiritual origins to become a scientifically validated practice for health and longevity. As researchers began to explore the effects of fasting on the body, they discovered its profound benefits. Studies have shown that fasting can improve insulin sensitivity, support cellular repair processes like autophagy, and even contribute to a longer lifespan.

Today, intermittent fasting has been tailored to fit into modern lifestyles, offering flexibility and customization to suit individual needs. While its ancient origins are rooted in survival and spirituality, intermittent fasting now serves as a bridge between past wisdom and modern science. It's a practice that empowers women, especially those over 60, to reclaim their health, embrace vitality, and step confidently into a new era of wellness.

In this book, we'll guide you through this timeless yet scientifically advanced practice, showing you how to make it work for your unique body and lifestyle.

Why Fasting Is Particularly Effective for Women Over 60

As women enter their 60s, their bodies undergo significant changes that make intermittent fasting an especially effective approach to health and well-being. At this stage in life, metabolic rates slow, hormonal balances shift, and maintaining a healthy weight often becomes more challenging. Intermittent fasting addresses these challenges with a unique set of benefits tailored to the needs of women over 60.

1. Supporting a Slower Metabolism

A slower metabolism is a natural part of aging, which can make it more difficult to burn calories efficiently. Intermittent fasting can help reignite the body's fat-burning potential by optimizing metabolic processes. During fasting periods, the body switches from using glucose as its primary energy source to burning stored fat. This metabolic shift not only aids weight management but also helps reduce visceral fat, particularly important for heart health and overall well-being.

2. Enhancing Insulin Sensitivity

As women age, they may become more prone to insulin resistance, which can increase the risk of type 2 diabetes. Intermittent fasting helps to stabilize blood sugar levels and improve insulin sensitivity by reducing the frequency of insulin spikes. By giving the body regular breaks from processing food, fasting allows the pancreas to reset and function more effectively, promoting healthier glucose metabolism.

3. Hormonal Balance and Post-Menopausal Health

The hormonal changes that occur after menopause, particularly the decline in estrogen levels, can affect everything from bone density to cardiovascular health. Intermittent fasting supports post-menopausal women by triggering cellular repair processes like autophagy, where the body removes damaged cells and regenerates healthier ones. This process has been linked to improved hormonal balance, reduced inflammation, and better overall health. Additionally, fasting has been shown to positively affect growth hormone levels, which naturally decrease with age. Increased growth hormone production can support muscle preservation, fat loss, and skin health, helping women feel more vibrant and youthful.

4. Combating Chronic Inflammation

Inflammation often increases with age and is linked to a variety of age-related diseases, including arthritis, heart disease, and cognitive decline. Intermittent fasting helps combat inflammation by reducing oxidative stress and improving the body's ability to repair damaged cells. This can lead to better joint health, reduced pain, and improved mental clarity: key priorities for women in their 60s and beyond.

5. Simplifying Healthy Living

One of the most attractive aspects of intermittent fasting for women over 60 is its simplicity. Unlike restrictive diets or calorie-counting programs, fasting doesn't require constant monitoring or meal preparation. With intermittent fasting, you can adapt the approach to suit your lifestyle, allowing you to enjoy food without the stress of constant dieting. This flexibility can make healthy living feel more achievable and less burdensome, especially in retirement or during busy family-oriented schedules.

6. Promoting Longevity and Vitality

The science of fasting aligns closely with the quest for longevity. Research suggests that fasting activates pathways in the body linked to a longer and healthier life. Processes like autophagy, reduced insulin levels, and improved cardiovascular health collectively contribute to a body that ages more gracefully. For women over 60, fasting offers a powerful way to embrace this stage of life with vitality and resilience.

A Practice Designed for Your Needs

Intermittent fasting is more than just a tool for weight loss: it's a holistic practice that can improve energy levels, support mental clarity, and enhance physical health. For women over 60, it offers a chance to rediscover control over their bodies, build healthier habits, and enjoy the golden years with confidence and vitality. This book will guide you in tailoring fasting to your unique needs, empowering you to unlock its incredible potential and live your best life.

What to Expect from This Book

This book is your comprehensive guide to intermittent fasting, tailored specifically for women over 60. Whether you're completely new to fasting or looking to deepen your understanding, you'll find the information, tools, and encouragement you need to succeed. Here's what you can expect to discover:

1. A Clear and Accessible Introduction to Intermittent Fasting

We'll start by breaking down what intermittent fasting is, how it works, and why it's particularly effective for women over 60. You'll gain a strong understanding of the science behind fasting and its benefits, all explained in simple, practical terms.

2. Personalized Guidance for Women Over 60

Your body is unique, especially at this stage of life. This book focuses on the specific needs, challenges, and opportunities that come with aging.

From managing hormonal changes to improving energy levels, we'll explore how intermittent fasting can be tailored to support your health and vitality.

3. Practical Advice to Get Started

Starting something new can feel overwhelming, but don't worry: we've got you covered. You'll find step-by-step guidance on how to begin fasting, choose the method that's right for you, and gradually build your confidence. We'll also cover how to handle common obstacles and make adjustments that suit your lifestyle.

4. A Focus on Holistic Wellness

Intermittent fasting is more than just a way to lose weight: it's a lifestyle that promotes overall health. This book integrates fasting with other wellness practices, such as balanced nutrition, gentle exercise, stress management, and better sleep. Together, these elements will help you achieve sustainable, long-term results.

5. Real-Life Inspiration and Success Stories

Sometimes the best motivation comes from others who've walked the same path. Throughout the book, you'll find stories of women over 60 who have transformed their lives with intermittent fasting. Their experiences will inspire and reassure you that it's never too late to make positive changes.

6. Delicious Recipes and Meal Ideas

Eating well during and after your fasting periods is essential for your success. This book includes simple, nutritious, and delicious recipes designed to support your body while keeping meal preparation easy and enjoyable.

7. Answers to Your Most Pressing Questions

From concerns about safety to practical tips for sticking with a fasting schedule, this book addresses the most common questions women over 60 have about intermittent fasting. By the end, you'll feel confident and informed about every aspect of the practice.

8. A Roadmap to Longevity and Confidence

This isn't just a guide to intermittent fasting: it's a roadmap to reclaiming your health, energy, and self-confidence. With the tools and strategies in this book, you'll be empowered to embrace the years ahead with strength, grace, and enthusiasm.

What You Won't Find

This is not a book about extreme dieting, unrealistic promises, or quick fixes. Instead, it's about sustainable, science-backed strategies that honor and respect the needs of your body as it ages.

By the time you finish this book, you'll have all the knowledge and tools you need to make intermittent fasting a natural and enjoyable part of your life. More importantly, you'll be equipped to embrace this new era of wellness with confidence, knowing that your best years are still ahead of you.

The Journey to Holistic Wellness

The Importance of Good Health at 60 and Beyond

Reaching your 60s is a milestone that comes with its own unique challenges and opportunities for health and well-being. While aging is a natural process, how you care for your body and mind can have a profound impact on the quality of life you experience during these years. Maintaining good health at this stage is not just about preventing disease; it is about living with vitality, joy, and independence.

Embracing the Changes of Aging

As you age, your body undergoes changes in metabolism, muscle mass, bone density, and hormonal balance. These shifts may feel like obstacles, but they are also invitations to adopt new habits that support your evolving needs. This is where a holistic approach to health becomes essential. Instead of focusing solely on weight or appearance, it is important to prioritize overall wellness, including physical strength, mental clarity, and emotional balance.

Reducing the Risk of Chronic Illness

After 60, the risk of developing chronic conditions such as heart disease, diabetes, and arthritis increases. However, many of these illnesses can be managed or even prevented with the right lifestyle choices. Intermittent fasting, combined with balanced nutrition and regular movement, offers a proven strategy for improving cardiovascular health, regulating blood sugar levels, and reducing inflammation. Taking control of your health now can help you enjoy more active and fulfilling years.

Supporting Mental and Emotional Well-Being

Good health is not just about the body. Mental clarity, emotional resilience, and a positive outlook are equally important. Intermittent fasting has been linked to improved cognitive function, mood stabilization, and even protection against age-related memory decline. By adopting practices that nurture both your body and mind, you can stay sharp, focused, and emotionally grounded.

Maintaining Independence and Quality of Life

As we age, one of the greatest fears is losing independence. Maintaining strength, mobility, and energy allows you to stay active and continue doing the things you love, whether it's playing with grandchildren, traveling, or pursuing hobbies. Good health also reduces the reliance on medications and medical interventions, giving you greater control over your daily life.

Investing in Longevity and Vitality

Your 60s and beyond are not the time to slow down; they are an opportunity to thrive. Focusing on your health now is an investment in your future. The choices you make today can help you avoid common pitfalls of aging, extend your lifespan, and ensure those years are full of vitality and purpose.

By committing to a journey of holistic wellness, you are choosing to make the most of this rewarding phase of life. This book will guide you in adopting sustainable, science-backed practices like intermittent fasting to help you feel your best, both now and for many years to come.

How Fasting Can Improve Energy, Vitality, and Quality of Life

Intermittent fasting is not just a tool for managing weight; it has a transformative effect on energy levels, vitality, and overall quality of life. By allowing the body to function more efficiently and promoting a state of balance, fasting can help you feel stronger, more focused, and ready to embrace life with renewed enthusiasm.

1. Boosting Natural Energy

One of the most immediate benefits of fasting is a noticeable increase in energy. During fasting periods, the body transitions from relying on glucose for fuel to burning stored fat. This process, known as ketosis, provides a steady and sustainable source of energy, reducing the mid-afternoon crashes and fatigue often associated with blood sugar fluctuations.

Fasting also reduces inflammation and oxidative stress, which are common culprits behind low energy in people over 60. By giving your body time to repair and rejuvenate, fasting helps you wake up feeling refreshed and stay active throughout the day.

2. Enhancing Mental Clarity and Focus

The brain thrives during fasting periods. Studies show that fasting increases the production of brain-derived neurotrophic factor (BDNF), a protein that supports brain health and cognitive function. This can lead to improved memory, sharper focus, and a greater sense of mental clarity.

For women over 60, maintaining cognitive health is a top priority, and fasting provides a natural way to support the brain's ability to stay sharp and adaptable as you age. Whether you're tackling a favorite hobby, learning something new, or simply enjoying a conversation, fasting can help you stay mentally engaged.

3. Improving Physical Vitality

Fasting triggers a powerful process called autophagy, where the body clears out damaged cells and replaces them with healthier ones. This cellular "clean-up" contributes to better muscle function, improved joint health, and greater overall physical vitality.

Many women over 60 find it challenging to maintain muscle mass and bone strength, but fasting combined with proper nutrition supports these areas by promoting the production of human growth hormone (HGH), which helps preserve muscle and keep you feeling strong and agile.

4. Stabilizing Mood and Emotional Balance

Mood swings and feelings of stress can become more common as we age, but fasting has been shown to stabilize mood by regulating hormones and reducing inflammation in the brain. Balanced blood sugar levels during fasting also help prevent the irritability or anxiety that can result from spikes and crashes in glucose.

This sense of emotional balance can lead to greater resilience in handling life's challenges, as well as a more optimistic outlook that enhances your overall quality of life.

5. Increasing Longevity and Purpose

Fasting is not only about feeling good today; it is about ensuring that you can maintain your vitality for years to come. By improving cellular health, regulating metabolism, and supporting the body's natural repair processes, fasting promotes longevity and reduces the risk of age-related diseases.

When you feel strong, energized, and mentally clear, you are better able to pursue the activities and relationships that bring you joy. This renewed sense of purpose and engagement adds depth and meaning to life, helping you make the most of every day.

A Path to Thriving, Not Just Surviving

Intermittent fasting empowers you to take control of your energy, vitality, and well-being in a way that feels natural and sustainable. By incorporating fasting into your life, you're not just making a dietary change, you're choosing to thrive, embrace new opportunities, and live with a renewed sense of vibrancy and purpose. This journey is about unlocking your full potential and enjoying a fulfilling life at 60 and beyond.

Chapter One

Understanding Intermittent Fasting

What Is Intermittent Fasting?

Definition and Core Principles

Intermittent fasting is a structured eating pattern that alternates between periods of eating and fasting. Unlike traditional diets that focus on what you eat, intermittent fasting emphasizes when you eat, giving your body extended breaks from food to trigger powerful healing and metabolic processes.

At its core, intermittent fasting is not about deprivation or extreme calorie restriction. Instead, it is a natural and flexible approach to eating that allows the body to function more efficiently. During fasting periods, the body stops focusing on digestion and shifts its energy toward repairing cells, burning fat, and regulating hormones.

The core principles of intermittent fasting include:

Eating within a specific time window: This could range from a daily 16-hour fast with an 8-hour eating window (known as the 16/8 method) to fasting for an entire day once or twice a week (the 5:2 method).

Giving the body time to reset: During fasting periods, insulin levels drop, and the body begins to burn stored fat for energy. At the same time, processes like cellular repair and detoxification are activated, promoting overall health.

Flexibility: Intermittent fasting can be adapted to fit your lifestyle, making it easier to maintain in the long term compared to restrictive diets.

Intermittent fasting is more than just a tool for weight loss. It is a practice deeply rooted in science that supports overall well-being by harmonizing with the body's natural rhythms. For women over 60, it offers a sustainable and effective way to reclaim health and vitality without the stress of complicated meal plans or calorie counting.

Scientifically Backed Benefits

Intermittent fasting is not just a trend, it is a scientifically supported practice with a wide range of benefits for overall health and well-being. Over the past few decades, numerous studies have highlighted the positive effects of fasting on the body and mind. For women over 60, these benefits are particularly compelling.

One of the key advantages of fasting is its ability to **regulate blood sugar levels**. Studies have shown that fasting helps improve insulin sensitivity, reducing the risk of type 2 diabetes. By giving the body breaks from constant digestion, insulin levels decrease, and the body becomes more efficient at processing glucose, preventing harmful spikes and crashes in blood sugar.

Fasting has also been proven to **reduce inflammation**. Chronic inflammation is linked to many age-related conditions, such as arthritis, heart disease, and even cognitive decline. Research indicates that fasting lowers markers of inflammation, allowing the body to heal and repair itself more effectively.

Another exciting area of research is fasting's impact on **cellular repair and longevity**. During fasting periods, the body triggers a process called **autophagy**, where it breaks down and recycles damaged or dysfunctional cells. This natural "clean-up" process is believed to play a critical role in slowing down the aging process and reducing the risk of diseases like cancer and Alzheimer's.

In terms of brain health, studies suggest that intermittent fasting increases levels of **brain-derived neurotrophic factor (BDNF)**, a protein that supports the growth and survival of neurons. This can enhance memory, focus, and cognitive function, offering protection against age-related mental decline.

Finally, intermittent fasting has been shown to support **weight management** and promote fat loss, particularly around the midsection. Unlike traditional diets that can lead to muscle loss, fasting helps preserve lean muscle while encouraging the body to burn stored fat for energy. This makes it an ideal strategy for maintaining strength and a healthy body composition as you age.

The evidence is clear: intermittent fasting is a powerful, science-backed tool for improving health, enhancing energy, and promoting longevity.

For women over 60, it offers a natural and effective way to feel stronger, sharper, and more vibrant at every stage of life.

How Fasting Works

The Biological Processes: Ketosis, Autophagy, and Insulin Regulation

Intermittent fasting is not just about eating less; it is about activating powerful biological processes that help your body function at its best. When you fast, your body undergoes several important changes that improve energy, repair cells, and balance hormones. Three of the most significant processes involved are ketosis, autophagy, and insulin regulation.

Ketosis is one of the first metabolic shifts that occurs during fasting. Normally, your body relies on glucose from the food you eat as its primary energy source. When you fast, your glucose reserves deplete, and your body begins to tap into its fat stores for fuel. This process produces molecules called ketones, which are used as an alternative energy source by your muscles and brain. Ketosis not only supports fat burning but also provides a steady, efficient source of energy, helping you feel more focused and energized during fasting periods.

Autophagy is another crucial process triggered by fasting. The term "autophagy" literally means "self-eating," and it refers to your body's natural ability to clean up and recycle damaged cells. During fasting, your body identifies old or malfunctioning cells, breaks them down, and uses their components to create new, healthy cells. This cellular renewal process is vital for maintaining overall health, slowing down the aging process, and reducing the risk of diseases like cancer and neurodegenerative conditions. Autophagy is particularly important for women over 60 because it helps counteract the effects of aging by keeping your cells functioning at their best.

Another key benefit of fasting is its role in **insulin regulation**. Insulin is a hormone that helps your body manage blood sugar levels by signaling cells to absorb glucose from your bloodstream. Over time, frequent eating and a diet high in refined carbohydrates can lead to insulin resistance, where your cells stop responding effectively to insulin. This can increase your risk of type 2 diabetes and other metabolic disorders. Fasting gives your body a break from constant insulin production, allowing insulin levels to drop and your cells to become more sensitive to its effects. This improved insulin sensitivity helps stabilize blood sugar levels, reduces fat storage, and promotes better overall metabolic health.

Together, ketosis, autophagy, and insulin regulation create a powerful synergy that supports your body's natural ability to heal, restore, and thrive. These processes are particularly beneficial for women over 60, helping to combat age-related metabolic changes, reduce inflammation, and enhance physical and cognitive vitality. Fasting is not just about skipping meals; it is about allowing your body to work more efficiently, unlocking its potential for improved health and well-being.

Why Fasting Works Better for Mature Women

Intermittent fasting can be particularly effective for mature women because it aligns with the natural changes that occur in the body as we age. These changes, such as shifts in metabolism, hormonal balance, and cellular function, make fasting not only beneficial but also uniquely suited to address the health challenges faced by women over 60.

As women age, their **metabolic rate naturally slows**, which means the body burns fewer calories at rest. This metabolic slowdown can lead to gradual weight gain, particularly around the midsection, even if eating habits remain the same. Intermittent fasting helps counteract this effect by promoting fat-burning through ketosis. By giving the body regular breaks from food, fasting encourages it to use stored fat for energy, making it easier to manage weight and reduce stubborn belly fat.

Hormonal shifts after menopause also play a significant role in how fasting benefits mature women. With the decline of estrogen levels, the body becomes more prone to storing fat and less efficient at metabolizing carbohydrates. These changes can increase the risk of insulin resistance and other metabolic conditions. Intermittent fasting helps stabilize blood sugar levels and improve insulin sensitivity, offering a powerful tool to address these hormonal challenges. By regulating insulin, fasting also reduces the risk of type 2 diabetes, which becomes more prevalent with age.

In addition to its metabolic benefits, fasting supports **cellular health and repair** through autophagy. This process is particularly important for women over 60 because cellular renewal slows down with age. As damaged cells accumulate, they can contribute to chronic inflammation and age-related diseases. Fasting activates autophagy, giving the body a chance to remove these dysfunctional cells and replace them with healthier ones. This helps combat inflammation, improve energy levels, and reduce the risk of illnesses such as heart disease and Alzheimer's.

Intermittent fasting also enhances **mental clarity and focus**, which can decline with age due to changes in brain function. Fasting increases the production of brain-derived neurotrophic factor (BDNF), a protein that supports brain health and neuroplasticity. This can help mature women stay sharp, improve memory, and reduce the risk of cognitive decline.

Finally, fasting aligns with the priorities and lifestyle of many women over 60. It simplifies eating habits by eliminating the need for strict calorie counting or complex meal plans, making it easier to maintain in the long term. Its flexibility allows women to adapt fasting schedules to their individual needs, social commitments, and energy levels, creating a sustainable approach to health and wellness.

Intermittent fasting works better for mature women because it addresses the specific challenges of aging. By targeting metabolism, hormones, and cellular repair, it provides a natural and effective way to enhance health, energy, and quality of life in this stage of life.

Types of Intermittent Fasting

The 16/8 Method

The 16/8 method is one of the most popular and beginner-friendly approaches to intermittent fasting. It involves fasting for 16 hours each day and eating all your meals within an 8-hour window. This method is particularly effective because it fits seamlessly into most lifestyles, allowing you to reap the benefits of fasting without drastically changing your daily routine.

How It Works

In the 16/8 method, you select an 8-hour period during which you consume all your meals and snacks. For example, you might choose to eat between **11:00 AM and 7:00 PM** or **12:00 PM and 8:00 PM**. Outside of this window, you fast, consuming only water, herbal teas, or black coffee to stay hydrated and support your body's fasting processes.

During the fasting period, your body depletes its glucose reserves and begins to burn stored fat for energy. This metabolic shift, known as ketosis, supports weight management and improves energy levels. The 8-hour eating window ensures you get enough nutrients and calories to fuel your day while giving your digestive system a much-needed break.

Why It's Ideal for Women Over 60

The 16/8 method is particularly well-suited for mature women because it balances simplicity with effectiveness. As women age, their bodies become more sensitive to long fasting periods. The 16-hour fasting window is long enough to trigger health benefits like fat burning, insulin regulation, and cellular repair, but short enough to avoid undue stress on the body.

This method also helps regulate blood sugar levels and reduce inflammation, two key factors in preventing age-related diseases. Additionally, by choosing an eating window that aligns with your natural rhythm, such as skipping breakfast or finishing dinner earlier, the 16/8 method is easy to incorporate into your daily routine without feeling overly restrictive.

Tips for Success

To maximize the benefits of the 16/8 method, focus on the quality of the food you eat during your eating window. Opt for nutrient-dense meals that include plenty of whole foods, lean proteins, healthy fats, and vegetables. Avoid overeating or consuming processed, sugary foods, as they can counteract the benefits of fasting.

Hydration is also essential during both the fasting and eating periods. Drinking water or herbal teas can help curb hunger and keep your body functioning optimally.

The 16/8 method is a powerful yet flexible way to embrace intermittent fasting. By giving your body regular breaks from eating, you can enhance your health, boost energy levels, and support longevity, all while enjoying a balanced and sustainable approach to eating. For women over 60, it offers a practical and effective strategy for feeling your best every day.

The 5:2 Method

The 5:2 method is a flexible and balanced approach to intermittent fasting that involves eating normally for five days of the week and significantly reducing calorie intake on the remaining two days. This method is particularly appealing for women over 60 because it allows for structured fasting without the need to fast every day, making it easier to maintain over the long term.

How It Works

With the 5:2 method, you choose two non-consecutive fasting days each week (for example, Monday and Thursday). On these fasting days, you limit your calorie intake to around **500–600 calories**, while the other five days are "normal eating" days.

The fasting days are not completely food-free. Instead, they involve mindful, low-calorie eating that focuses on nutrient-dense foods like vegetables, lean proteins, and healthy fats. This helps you stay satisfied and avoid feeling overly deprived.

During the fasting days, your body benefits from a temporary caloric deficit, which can promote fat loss, improve insulin sensitivity, and activate cellular repair processes like autophagy. On the non-fasting days, you can enjoy regular, balanced meals without strict restrictions, creating a sustainable rhythm of eating and fasting.

Why It's Ideal for Women Over 60

The 5:2 method works well for mature women because it provides flexibility and minimizes the stress that can come with longer or daily fasting periods. By fasting on just two days a week, you give your body time to rest and reset while still maintaining a regular routine on the other days.

This approach is also excellent for managing metabolic changes that occur after 60. The fasting days allow your body to stabilize blood sugar levels, promote fat-burning, and reduce inflammation. Meanwhile, the non-fasting days ensure you receive adequate nutrition to support your energy, bone health, and overall vitality.

Additionally, the 5:2 method can be adapted to fit your lifestyle. If you have a social event or a busy schedule on one of your planned fasting days, you can easily shift it to another day without disrupting your progress.

Tips for Success

On fasting days, focus on nutrient-dense, low-calorie meals that are high in fiber and protein. For example, a typical fasting day might include:

- A breakfast of boiled eggs and steamed spinach.
- A dinner of grilled chicken breast with a large mixed vegetable salad.

Hydration is key during fasting days. Drinking plenty of water, herbal teas, or even broths can help keep hunger at bay and support your body's natural detox processes.

On non-fasting days, avoid overindulging and aim for balanced meals that include whole grains, lean proteins, healthy fats, and fresh produce. This ensures your body gets the nutrients it needs to stay strong and energized throughout the week.

The 5:2 method is a simple yet effective way to practice intermittent fasting. It offers flexibility, long-term sustainability, and significant health benefits without requiring daily fasting. For women over 60, it provides a practical framework to enhance health, improve energy, and support a more vibrant life.

Alternate-Day Fasting

Alternate-day fasting is an intermittent fasting method that involves alternating between days of fasting and days of regular eating. On fasting days, calorie intake is drastically reduced, while non-fasting days allow for normal, unrestricted eating. This method is known for its simplicity and effectiveness in promoting fat loss, improving metabolic health, and supporting cellular repair.

How It Works

With alternate-day fasting, you alternate between two types of days:

- **Fasting days**: Calorie intake is limited to around 500–600 calories, typically consumed in one or two light meals.
- **Eating days**: No restrictions are placed on the amount or type of food you eat, allowing for a balanced and enjoyable diet.

This schedule allows your body to regularly experience the benefits of fasting without requiring extended periods of food deprivation. On fasting days, the body taps into stored fat for energy, reduces insulin levels, and activates processes like autophagy. On eating days, you replenish nutrients and enjoy the foods you love, making this method easier to sustain over time.

Why It's Effective for Women Over 60

Alternate-day fasting is particularly effective for mature women because it combines the metabolic benefits of fasting with the flexibility of regular eating days. This balance allows women over 60 to experience significant health improvements without feeling restricted or fatigued.

One of the primary advantages of this method is its impact on **weight management and fat loss**, especially in areas like the abdomen where fat tends to accumulate after menopause. By alternating between fasting and eating days, the body consistently cycles between fat-burning and metabolic recovery, leading to sustainable weight loss.

Additionally, the frequent fasting periods help improve **insulin sensitivity** and regulate blood sugar levels, both of which are crucial for preventing age-related conditions such as type 2 diabetes. The method also supports cardiovascular health by lowering cholesterol and reducing inflammation, which are common concerns for women over 60.

Alternate-day fasting is a powerful tool for promoting **cellular health and longevity**. The regular activation of autophagy helps the body eliminate damaged cells and replace them with healthier ones, reducing the risk of chronic diseases and slowing the aging process.

Tips for Success

To make alternate-day fasting manageable, it is essential to plan your meals and stay hydrated. On fasting days, focus on low-calorie, nutrient-dense foods that keep you feeling full, such as:

- A vegetable soup with lean protein like chicken or tofu.
- A salad with plenty of greens, a drizzle of olive oil, and a small portion of nuts or seeds.

Hydration is key to curbing hunger and maintaining energy levels on fasting days. Drink water, herbal teas, or black coffee to support your body during the fast.

On eating days, aim for a balanced diet rich in whole foods. While you can enjoy more flexibility on these days, it is still important to prioritize nutritious meals that fuel your body and support your overall health goals.

Sustainability and Flexibility

Alternate-day fasting offers a flexible approach to fasting that can be easily adapted to your lifestyle. If fasting every other day feels too intense at first, you can start with modified versions, such as fasting only two or three days a week. This gradual approach allows you to build confidence and adjust to the rhythm of fasting.

For women over 60, alternate-day fasting provides a structured yet adaptable strategy for enhancing health, improving energy, and promoting longevity. By alternating between fasting and regular eating, this method empowers you to embrace a healthier lifestyle without sacrificing the foods and experiences you enjoy.

The 24-Hour Method and OMAD (One Meal a Day)

The 24-hour fasting method and OMAD (One Meal a Day) are two advanced approaches to intermittent fasting. These methods involve extending fasting periods to a full 24 hours or limiting daily food intake to a single meal. While more challenging than other fasting methods, they offer significant benefits for women over 60 who are ready to take their fasting practice to the next level.

How the 24-Hour Method Works

The 24-hour fasting method involves fasting from one meal to the same meal the following day. For example, if you eat dinner at 6:00 PM, your next meal would be dinner at 6:00 PM the following day. During the fasting period, you consume only water, herbal teas, or black coffee.

This method is typically practiced one or two times per week and provides a longer fasting window that allows the body to fully enter fat-burning mode, stabilize insulin levels, and activate autophagy. On non-fasting days, you return to regular eating patterns, ensuring you meet your nutritional needs.

How OMAD (One Meal a Day) Works

OMAD, or One Meal a Day, is a variation of the 24-hour fasting method where you consume all your daily calories within a single meal. Unlike the strict 24-hour fast, OMAD typically includes a daily eating window of about one hour. For example, you might choose to eat dinner every day at 6:00 PM and fast for the remaining 23 hours.

The meal in OMAD should be nutrient-dense and balanced, providing your body with enough calories, protein, healthy fats, and carbohydrates to sustain energy and support health. While challenging, OMAD simplifies meal planning and creates a strong calorie deficit, which can be highly effective for weight loss and metabolic improvements.

Why These Methods Are Effective for Women Over 60

The extended fasting periods in the 24-hour method and OMAD amplify many of the health benefits associated with shorter fasting windows. These include:

- **Enhanced fat burning**: With a prolonged fasting period, the body has more time to use stored fat for energy, which can help reduce stubborn fat deposits often accumulated after menopause.
- **Improved insulin sensitivity**: Longer fasts provide extended breaks for the body to regulate blood sugar levels and improve insulin function, reducing the risk of type 2 diabetes.
- **Deep cellular repair**: Extended fasting enhances autophagy, promoting the cleanup of damaged cells and supporting the body's natural anti-aging processes.
- **Mental clarity**: Many people report heightened focus and mental sharpness during longer fasting periods due to the increased production of ketones, which serve as a clean and efficient energy source for the brain.

Tips for Success

For the 24-hour method or OMAD, preparation and balance are key. Here are some tips to make these methods sustainable:

- **Start gradually**: If you are new to fasting, build up to these methods by starting with shorter fasting windows, such as the 16/8 or 5:2 methods.
- **Focus on nutrient-dense meals**: When breaking your fast, ensure your meal is rich in lean proteins, healthy fats, and fiber. Avoid processed or sugary foods that can disrupt the benefits of fasting.

- **Stay hydrated**: Drinking plenty of water, herbal teas, or broth during fasting periods is essential to prevent dehydration and keep energy levels stable.
- **Listen to your body**: Longer fasting periods can be challenging, so pay attention to how you feel. If you experience dizziness, extreme fatigue, or other concerning symptoms, consider shortening the fast or consulting a healthcare provider.

Sustainability and Flexibility

While the 24-hour method and OMAD can deliver significant results, they may not be suitable for everyone to practice regularly. Women over 60 may prefer to use these methods occasionally, as a way to deepen their fasting practice or reset their eating habits after holidays or indulgent periods.

Both approaches offer powerful health benefits, but they require careful planning and attention to nutrition to avoid potential downsides, such as nutrient deficiencies or fatigue. For those who are ready to embrace a more advanced fasting strategy, the 24-hour method and OMAD provide an effective way to enhance health, support weight management, and promote longevity.

Tips for Choosing the Right Method

With so many intermittent fasting methods available, it's important to choose the one that best fits your lifestyle, health goals, and personal preferences. The key to success with intermittent fasting is sustainability—selecting a method that you can comfortably stick to in the long term. Here are some tips to help you decide:

1. Start Simple

If you are new to intermittent fasting, begin with an approachable method like the 16/8. This option is easy to integrate into your daily routine and allows you to adjust to fasting without feeling overwhelmed. Once you are comfortable, you can experiment with more advanced methods like the 5:2 or alternate-day fasting.

2. Consider Your Lifestyle

Think about your daily schedule, social commitments, and energy needs. For example, if you enjoy having breakfast with family or dinner with friends, the 16/8 or OMAD methods may be more practical than alternate-day fasting. If you prefer more flexibility, the 5:2 method lets you choose fasting days that work best for your week.

3. Align with Your Health Goals

Your goals will help determine the best fasting method for you:

- If you're looking to lose weight, methods like the 16/8 or 5:2 are highly effective while still allowing for a balanced lifestyle.
- For deeper metabolic benefits, such as reducing inflammation or improving insulin sensitivity, alternate-day fasting or the 24-hour method might be more suitable.
- If simplicity is your priority, OMAD provides a straightforward way to manage your meals.

4. Listen to Your Body

Pay attention to how you feel during fasting periods. If a method leaves you overly fatigued, irritable, or hungry, it may not be the right fit. Your body's signals are important indicators of what works and what doesn't. It's okay to switch methods or make adjustments as needed.

5. Adapt Over Time

Your needs and preferences may change, and so can your fasting method. Some women prefer to start with shorter fasting windows and gradually extend them as their bodies adapt. Others find that alternating between methods, such as combining 16/8 during the week with occasional 24-hour fasts, keeps things interesting and effective.

6. Consult a Healthcare Professional

If you have any pre-existing medical conditions, such as diabetes or cardiovascular issues, consult your doctor before starting a fasting regimen. They can help you choose a method that is safe and aligned with your health needs.

Intermittent fasting is not a one-size-fits-all approach. The best method is the one that supports your health, fits your lifestyle, and makes you feel strong and empowered. By starting with a method that feels achievable and adapting as needed, you can create a fasting routine that becomes a natural and enjoyable part of your life.

Chapter Two

Why Intermittent Fasting Is Ideal for Women Over 60

The Evolving Body

Hormonal Changes After Menopause

Menopause marks a significant transition in a woman's life, bringing about profound hormonal changes that affect the body in many ways. After menopause, the production of key hormones such as estrogen and progesterone decreases dramatically, leading to shifts in metabolism, fat distribution, and overall energy levels. These changes can create challenges, but they also present opportunities to adopt new habits, like intermittent fasting, that align with the body's evolving needs.

One of the most noticeable effects of post-menopausal hormonal shifts is a **slower metabolism**. Estrogen plays a crucial role in regulating how the body stores and burns fat. As estrogen levels decline, the body becomes more prone to storing fat, particularly in the abdominal area, and less efficient at breaking it down. This can lead to weight gain even when eating habits remain unchanged. Intermittent fasting helps counteract this process by promoting fat burning through ketosis and improving overall metabolic efficiency.

Another common issue after menopause is **increased insulin resistance**, which occurs when the body becomes less responsive to insulin, the hormone that regulates blood sugar. This can lead to blood sugar fluctuations, energy crashes, and a higher risk of developing type 2 diabetes. Fasting supports insulin sensitivity by giving the body a break from constant digestion, allowing insulin levels to stabilize and glucose to be processed more effectively.

Hormonal changes can also contribute to **chronic inflammation**, a condition linked to a variety of age-related health issues such as arthritis, heart disease, and cognitive decline. By reducing inflammation markers, intermittent fasting promotes a healthier internal environment, helping to mitigate some of the negative effects of hormonal imbalance.

Finally, declining estrogen levels can affect **mental clarity and mood stability**, often leading to brain fog, irritability, or even depression. Fasting has been shown to enhance brain function by increasing the production of brain-derived neurotrophic factor (BDNF), a protein that supports cognitive health and emotional balance.

While hormonal changes after menopause can feel like obstacles, they are not insurmountable. Intermittent fasting provides a practical and effective way to address these challenges, helping women over 60 maintain a healthy weight, stabilize energy levels, and support overall well-being during this new phase of life.

The Effects of Aging on Metabolism, Muscles, and Body Fat

As women age, their bodies naturally undergo changes that affect metabolism, muscle mass, and fat distribution. These shifts are part of the aging process, but they can pose challenges to maintaining health and vitality. Understanding these changes and how intermittent fasting can address them is key to feeling strong and confident in your 60s and beyond.

Metabolism

One of the most significant changes with age is a slowing metabolism. The body burns fewer calories at rest, which means that maintaining a stable weight becomes more difficult. This decline in metabolic rate is influenced by hormonal changes, a natural reduction in muscle mass, and a decrease in physical activity levels.

A slower metabolism can lead to weight gain over time, particularly in the form of increased fat storage. Intermittent fasting helps counteract this by promoting fat burning through ketosis, a metabolic state where the body uses stored fat for energy. Fasting also improves metabolic flexibility, making it easier for your body to switch between burning carbs and fats, which supports efficient energy use and weight management.

Muscle Mass

After the age of 30, muscle mass naturally begins to decline in a process called sarcopenia. By the time women reach their 60s, this loss of muscle can contribute to decreased strength, reduced mobility, and a slower metabolism, as muscles play a critical role in calorie burning.

Intermittent fasting, combined with resistance exercises and adequate protein intake during eating periods, can help preserve muscle mass. Fasting stimulates the production of human growth hormone (HGH), which supports muscle maintenance and repair. This is particularly important for staying active, maintaining independence, and preventing injuries as you age.

Body Fat

With aging, fat distribution tends to shift, particularly after menopause. Women often experience an increase in abdominal fat, which poses a greater health risk than fat stored in other areas. Visceral fat, the type of fat stored around internal organs, is linked to inflammation, insulin resistance, and cardiovascular disease.

Intermittent fasting is highly effective in reducing visceral fat. By extending the time between meals, the body depletes its glycogen stores and begins burning fat for energy. This not only helps with weight loss but also reduces the harmful fat that contributes to chronic health issues.

A Balanced Approach

The combined effects of a slower metabolism, declining muscle mass, and changes in fat distribution can feel frustrating, but they are not inevitable. Intermittent fasting provides a powerful way to address these challenges by optimizing how your body uses energy, supporting muscle health, and targeting fat stores.

By incorporating fasting into your lifestyle and pairing it with regular physical activity and a nutrient-dense diet, you can mitigate the effects of aging and maintain a strong, healthy, and energized body for years to come.

The Long-Term Health Benefits of Fasting

Weight Management

Maintaining a healthy weight becomes increasingly challenging as women age, particularly after 60, due to a slower metabolism, hormonal changes, and shifts in fat distribution. Intermittent fasting offers a natural and effective solution for weight management by optimizing the body's energy use and encouraging fat loss without the need for restrictive diets or calorie counting.

One of the key ways fasting supports weight control is by promoting **fat-burning through ketosis**. During fasting periods, the body uses up its glycogen (stored glucose) reserves and begins to burn stored fat for energy. This metabolic shift not only helps reduce overall body fat but also targets visceral fat, the type of fat stored around internal organs that poses significant health risks.

Intermittent fasting also helps regulate **appetite and hunger hormones**. As the eating schedule becomes more structured, the production of ghrelin (the hunger hormone) stabilizes, reducing cravings and overeating. Many women find that fasting helps them regain control over their eating habits, making it easier to resist unhealthy snacks and avoid mindless eating.

Another important aspect is fasting's ability to **balance insulin levels**, which plays a crucial role in weight regulation. Constant snacking and frequent meals can lead to chronically elevated insulin levels, promoting fat storage and increasing the risk of insulin resistance. Fasting provides the body with regular breaks from food, allowing insulin levels to drop and improving the body's ability to burn fat.

For women over 60, intermittent fasting is not just about weight loss, it's about sustainable weight management. It allows you to maintain a healthy weight while preserving muscle mass, improving energy levels, and reducing the risks associated with excess fat, such as heart disease and type 2 diabetes.

By focusing on a balanced approach that combines fasting with nutrient-rich meals during eating periods, you can achieve long-term weight control while feeling satisfied and energized. This approach empowers women to maintain a healthy body composition without the stress of extreme diets, ensuring that they feel strong, confident, and vibrant in their golden years.

Improving Cardiovascular Health

Cardiovascular health is a key concern for women over 60, as aging and hormonal changes can increase the risk of heart disease, high blood pressure, and other related conditions. Intermittent fasting offers a natural and effective way to support heart health by addressing many of the underlying factors that contribute to cardiovascular issues.

One of the most significant benefits of fasting is its ability to **reduce inflammation**, which is a major contributor to heart disease. Chronic inflammation damages blood vessels and increases the risk of plaque buildup, leading to conditions such as atherosclerosis. Studies show that intermittent fasting lowers markers of inflammation, helping to protect the cardiovascular system and improve overall heart health.

Fasting also plays a crucial role in **regulating blood pressure**, a common issue among older adults. By promoting better blood vessel function and reducing oxidative stress, fasting helps maintain healthy blood pressure levels, reducing strain on the heart and lowering the risk of stroke and other cardiovascular events.

Another important benefit is **improved cholesterol levels**. Intermittent fasting has been shown to decrease LDL (bad) cholesterol and triglycerides while increasing HDL (good) cholesterol. These changes help prevent the buildup of fatty deposits in the arteries, reducing the risk of blockages that can lead to heart attacks.

Additionally, fasting improves **insulin sensitivity**, which is closely linked to heart health. High insulin levels and insulin resistance can contribute to weight gain, high blood pressure, and increased cholesterol, all of which put additional strain on the heart. By stabilizing insulin levels, fasting reduces these risk factors, promoting a healthier cardiovascular system.

For women over 60, intermittent fasting offers a holistic approach to maintaining heart health. By addressing key risk factors such as inflammation, high blood pressure, and cholesterol imbalances, fasting supports a strong, resilient cardiovascular system, allowing you to live with greater vitality and peace of mind.

Combining fasting with other heart-healthy practices, such as regular physical activity, a balanced diet rich in fruits, vegetables, and healthy fats, and stress management techniques, further enhances its benefits. Together, these strategies empower women to protect their heart health and enjoy a longer, healthier life.

Preventing Type 2 Diabetes

Type 2 diabetes is a growing concern for women over 60, as aging, hormonal changes, and lifestyle factors can increase the risk of developing this condition. Intermittent fasting has emerged as a highly effective tool for reducing this risk by addressing some of the root causes of diabetes, including insulin resistance and unstable blood sugar levels.

When you practice intermittent fasting, your body has extended periods to rest from constantly processing food. This allows **insulin levels to decrease** and improves your cells' sensitivity to insulin. Insulin is a hormone responsible for helping glucose enter your cells for energy. Over time, poor dietary habits and frequent eating can lead to insulin resistance, where the cells stop responding effectively to insulin. Fasting gives the body an opportunity to reset, making insulin work more efficiently and helping maintain stable blood sugar levels.

Research has shown that intermittent fasting can significantly reduce **fasting blood sugar and hemoglobin A1c levels**, two key indicators of diabetes risk. By stabilizing blood sugar over time, fasting not only lowers the likelihood of developing type 2 diabetes but can also help manage it in individuals already diagnosed.

Another way fasting aids in diabetes prevention is by encouraging **weight loss and fat reduction**, particularly around the abdomen. Abdominal fat, or visceral fat, is closely linked to insulin resistance and increased blood sugar levels. Fasting helps the body burn this stored fat, improving overall metabolic health and reducing strain on the pancreas, the organ responsible for producing insulin.

For women over 60, fasting offers the added benefit of simplicity. Unlike complex meal plans or restrictive diets often recommended for blood sugar control, intermittent fasting focuses on timing rather than specific food restrictions. This makes it a sustainable, practical approach for managing health while still enjoying meals that fit your lifestyle.

By integrating intermittent fasting with healthy eating habits and regular physical activity, you can significantly lower your risk of type 2 diabetes while supporting your overall well-being. Fasting is not just about managing weight; it is a proactive step toward protecting your long-term health and maintaining independence as you age.

Promoting Longevity

One of the most compelling benefits of intermittent fasting is its potential to enhance longevity. As women enter their 60s and beyond, the focus often shifts from simply maintaining health to optimizing it for a longer, more vibrant life. Intermittent fasting has been shown to activate processes within the body that contribute to aging gracefully, reducing the risk of age-related diseases, and extending life expectancy.

At the heart of fasting's impact on longevity is a process called **autophagy**. During fasting periods, the body initiates this cellular "clean-up" mechanism, removing damaged or dysfunctional cells and replacing them with healthier ones. Autophagy helps to prevent the accumulation of cellular debris, which is associated with chronic inflammation, aging, and diseases such as cancer, Alzheimer's, and Parkinson's. By promoting cellular renewal, fasting keeps the body functioning optimally, supporting both physical and mental health over time.

Fasting also contributes to longevity by reducing **oxidative stress**, a key factor in the aging process. Oxidative stress occurs when there is an imbalance between free radicals (unstable molecules) and antioxidants in the body, leading to cellular damage. Intermittent fasting enhances the body's natural antioxidant defenses and minimizes the production of free radicals, protecting tissues and organs from premature aging.

Additionally, fasting supports longevity by improving **metabolic health**. Chronic conditions like type 2 diabetes, obesity, and cardiovascular disease can significantly shorten lifespan. Fasting addresses these risks by regulating insulin levels, reducing inflammation, and encouraging fat loss, particularly around the abdominal area where visceral fat poses the greatest health threats.

Another fascinating benefit of fasting is its ability to stimulate the production of **human growth hormone (HGH)**, a hormone that declines with age. HGH plays a vital role in cell repair, muscle maintenance, and overall vitality. By naturally boosting HGH levels, fasting helps the body stay strong and resilient as it ages.

For women over 60, intermittent fasting offers a realistic and accessible way to tap into these longevity-promoting mechanisms. It does not require extreme changes to diet or lifestyle, making it an adaptable approach to enhancing health and extending life.

By combining fasting with other healthy habits—such as regular exercise, stress management, and a diet rich in nutrient-dense foods—you can unlock the potential for a longer, healthier, and more fulfilling life. Intermittent fasting is not just about adding years to your life; it's about adding life to your years, empowering you to embrace the future with energy, clarity, and confidence.

Challenges and How to Overcome Them

Common Concerns: "Is It Safe for Me?"

For many women over 60, the first question about intermittent fasting is whether it's a safe and appropriate choice for their age and health status. This is a natural concern, as the body's needs change with time, and new practices should always be approached with caution. The good news is that intermittent fasting is generally safe for most healthy individuals, including women over 60, when done thoughtfully and tailored to their unique needs.

Understanding Your Body's Needs

As you age, your body becomes more sensitive to changes in diet and lifestyle. Factors like slower metabolism, decreased muscle mass, and possible chronic health conditions require a mindful approach to fasting. While intermittent fasting offers numerous benefits, it is essential to listen to your body and recognize that what works for others may need adjustment to suit your personal circumstances.

When to Exercise Caution

There are certain situations where fasting may not be appropriate or may require additional guidance. For example:

If you have existing health conditions such as diabetes, low blood pressure, or a history of eating disorders, consult a healthcare professional before starting.

If you take medications that must be taken with food, you may need to modify fasting periods.

If you experience fatigue or dizziness, consider shortening your fasting window or incorporating a less restrictive method like the 16/8 or 5:2 approach.

Tips for Fasting Safely

To ensure that fasting is safe and beneficial for you, consider these practical tips:

Start gradually: If you are new to fasting, begin with shorter fasting windows, such as 12 to 14 hours, and gradually increase the duration as your body adapts.

Stay hydrated: Drink plenty of water and herbal teas during fasting periods to prevent dehydration and support your body's natural functions.

Focus on nutrient-dense meals: During eating periods, prioritize whole, unprocessed foods rich in vitamins, minerals, and protein to provide the energy and nutrients your body needs.

Monitor how you feel: Pay attention to your energy levels, mood, and hunger cues. If you feel overly fatigued or unwell, adjust your fasting schedule or consult a healthcare provider.

Reassurance for Beginners

Scientific research and practical experience show that intermittent fasting can be a safe and effective practice for women over 60, particularly when approached with care and flexibility. The body is remarkably adaptable, and many women find that fasting improves their energy, digestion, and overall health after just a few weeks of practice.

If you're unsure about whether intermittent fasting is right for you, consider consulting your doctor or a nutritionist. A professional can help evaluate your health history, discuss potential risks, and recommend a fasting plan that aligns with your needs and goals.

Remember, the goal of intermittent fasting is not to force your body into a rigid routine but to support it in becoming healthier and more balanced. By starting with a personalized approach and staying attuned to your body's signals, you can enjoy the many benefits of fasting with confidence and peace of mind.

Specific Adjustments for Those with Chronic Conditions

Intermittent fasting can offer many benefits for overall health, but for women over 60 with chronic conditions, it is essential to approach fasting with caution and adapt it to their specific needs. Conditions such as diabetes, high blood pressure, or arthritis may require modifications to ensure fasting is both safe and effective. Here's how to navigate intermittent fasting while managing chronic health issues.

Fasting with Diabetes

For individuals with diabetes, especially type 2, intermittent fasting can help regulate blood sugar levels and improve insulin sensitivity. However, it's crucial to:

Work with your doctor: Before starting, consult your healthcare provider, as fasting can impact medication dosages, particularly for insulin or other glucose-lowering drugs.

Choose shorter fasting windows: Start with a method like the 16/8 approach, which provides periods of fasting while still allowing regular meals to manage blood sugar.

Monitor your blood sugar levels closely: Frequent checks can help you understand how fasting affects your glucose levels and avoid hypoglycemia or other complications.

Focus on balanced meals: During eating periods, prioritize foods that stabilize blood sugar, such as high-fiber vegetables, lean proteins, and healthy fats, while avoiding refined carbohydrates and sugars.

Fasting with High Blood Pressure

For women managing high blood pressure, intermittent fasting can help improve heart health and lower blood pressure by reducing inflammation and supporting weight loss. However, to ensure safety:

Stay hydrated: Dehydration during fasting can cause blood pressure fluctuations. Drink plenty of water and herbal teas during fasting periods.

Avoid excessive salt intake: On eating days, reduce sodium and prioritize potassium-rich foods like leafy greens, bananas, and avocados, which support heart health.

Monitor blood pressure regularly: Keep track of your readings to observe how fasting affects your condition and make adjustments if needed.

Fasting with Arthritis or Chronic Pain

For those with arthritis or chronic pain, intermittent fasting can reduce inflammation, potentially alleviating symptoms. To make fasting more effective:

Incorporate anti-inflammatory foods: During eating periods, focus on foods rich in omega-3 fatty acids (like salmon, walnuts, and flaxseeds) and antioxidants (such as berries, spinach, and turmeric).

Start with a moderate fasting method: A method like 5:2 or 16/8 is less stressful on the body and easier to sustain while managing chronic pain.

Stay physically active: Gentle exercises like yoga or swimming during fasting periods can improve joint mobility and reduce stiffness without overexertion.

General Guidelines for Fasting with Chronic Conditions

Consult a healthcare professional: Always discuss fasting plans with your doctor, especially if you take medications or have a medical history that could affect fasting.

Start slowly: Introduce fasting gradually to allow your body to adapt and to observe how it interacts with your condition.

Listen to your body: If you experience dizziness, weakness, or other adverse symptoms, adjust your fasting window or stop fasting and consult a professional.

Ensure balanced nutrition: During eating periods, focus on nutrient-dense meals to provide your body with the vitamins and minerals it needs to support your condition.

Intermittent fasting can be a powerful tool for improving health, even for women with chronic conditions. By making thoughtful adjustments and working closely with a healthcare provider, you can tailor fasting to your unique needs, helping you achieve better health and an improved quality of life.

Chapter Three

Getting Started with Intermittent Fasting

Preparing Mentally and Physically

Overcoming the Fear of Fasting

Starting something new can be intimidating, and intermittent fasting is no exception. Many women feel hesitant about fasting because it challenges long-held beliefs about eating habits, such as the idea that skipping meals is unhealthy or that hunger will be unbearable. The good news is that intermittent fasting is not about deprivation; it's about empowering your body to function optimally. By addressing common fears and understanding the process, you can overcome any apprehension and confidently begin your fasting journey.

Understanding Hunger

One of the most common fears about fasting is the worry that hunger will be too difficult to manage. While it's true that you may feel hungry at first, this sensation often decreases as your body adapts to fasting. Hunger comes in waves and is regulated by the hormone ghrelin, which naturally rises and falls throughout the day. With time, your body adjusts to the new eating schedule, and hunger becomes more manageable.

To ease this transition, stay hydrated and consider starting with shorter fasting periods, such as 12 to 14 hours, before gradually increasing the duration. Herbal teas, sparkling water, and black coffee can also help curb hunger and provide a sense of satisfaction during fasting periods.

Challenging Myths About Skipping Meals

Many people fear that skipping meals will harm their metabolism or cause muscle loss. However, scientific research shows that intermittent fasting, when done correctly, does not "damage" metabolism. In fact, it can boost metabolic flexibility, allowing your body to efficiently switch between burning glucose and fat for energy.

Concerns about muscle loss are also addressed through proper nutrition. During eating windows, focus on consuming adequate protein, healthy fats, and fiber to support muscle maintenance and overall health. Light resistance exercises can further help preserve and strengthen muscles as part of your routine.

Letting Go of Dieting Mindsets

If you've experienced restrictive dieting in the past, you might associate fasting with feelings of deprivation or failure. Intermittent fasting is different. It's not about counting calories or following rigid rules, it's about creating a sustainable pattern that works for you. By focusing on when to eat rather than what to eat, fasting simplifies your approach to food, reducing stress and encouraging mindfulness.

Building Confidence Through Knowledge

Fear often comes from the unknown. Learning about the science and benefits of fasting can help build confidence and dispel doubts. Understand that fasting is a natural process your body is designed for, and many women have successfully embraced this practice to improve their health and vitality.

Setting Realistic Expectations

It's natural to worry about "doing it wrong" or whether fasting will deliver results. Remember, intermittent fasting is not a race but a lifestyle adjustment. Progress may be gradual, but the benefits will come with consistency and patience.

Focus on Your Goals

Whenever doubts arise, remind yourself why you're embarking on this journey. Whether your goal is better energy, improved health, or a sense of control over your eating habits, keeping these motivations in mind can help you push past fear and take those first steps.

By approaching intermittent fasting with an open mind, realistic expectations, and a focus on progress rather than perfection, you can overcome fear and unlock the incredible benefits fasting has to offer. It's a journey of empowerment, not restriction, and one that can lead to a healthier, more confident you.

Creating a Positive Mindset

A positive mindset is one of the most important tools for successfully starting and maintaining intermittent fasting. Approaching this new lifestyle with optimism and confidence can make the transition smoother and help you stay motivated as you build healthier habits. Fasting is not just a physical practice; it's also a mental one that requires patience, self-compassion, and a focus on the benefits ahead.

Reframe Fasting as Self-Care

Rather than viewing fasting as something restrictive, think of it as an act of self-care. By giving your body time to rest and heal, you're supporting its natural ability to function at its best. Remind yourself that intermittent fasting is not about depriving yourself but about creating a healthier, more energized version of you.

Focus on the Benefits

Keeping your goals in mind can help you maintain a positive attitude. Whether you're fasting to improve energy levels, support weight management, or enhance your overall well-being, visualize the outcome you want to achieve. Write down your goals and revisit them regularly to stay motivated.

Start with Small Wins

Building confidence starts with achievable steps. Begin with a fasting method that feels manageable, such as the 16/8 approach or even a 12-hour fast, and gradually extend your fasting window as you grow more comfortable. Celebrating small wins along the way, like completing your first fasting period or noticing improved energy, reinforces your progress and helps you stay focused.

Replace Doubt with Curiosity

It's natural to have questions or doubts when trying something new. Instead of letting uncertainty hold you back, approach fasting with curiosity and a willingness to learn. Each fasting period is an opportunity to observe how your body responds, refine your approach, and discover what works best for you.

Practice Self-Compassion

Starting a new lifestyle change can come with challenges, and it's important to be kind to yourself during the process. If you experience setbacks, such as breaking a fast early or feeling unsure about your progress, remember that this is part of the journey. A positive mindset includes giving yourself grace and focusing on consistency rather than perfection.

Surround Yourself with Support

Positive reinforcement from others can be incredibly motivating. Share your goals with supportive friends or family members, or consider joining an online community of women practicing intermittent fasting. Hearing about others' experiences and successes can inspire you and provide valuable insights.

Visualize Success

Take a moment each day to visualize yourself thriving with fasting. Picture the energy, confidence, and health improvements you'll gain as you commit to this lifestyle. Visualization helps to reinforce your belief in your ability to succeed and makes your goals feel more tangible.

By creating a positive mindset, you set the foundation for long-term success with intermittent fasting. This mental shift not only makes fasting more enjoyable but also empowers you to embrace this journey with confidence and enthusiasm. Your outlook matters, and with the right mindset, you can turn fasting into a fulfilling and transformative part of your life.

How to Personalize Fasting

Assessing Your Health

Before starting intermittent fasting, it's important to evaluate your current health to ensure the approach you choose aligns with your body's needs and capabilities. A thorough understanding of your physical condition helps you tailor fasting to suit your unique circumstances and maximize its benefits.

Consult Your Healthcare Provider

If you have any pre-existing medical conditions, take medications, or are unsure about whether fasting is right for you, consult your healthcare provider. They can help you determine if fasting is safe and recommend specific modifications based on your medical history. Conditions such as diabetes, hypertension, or digestive issues may require adjustments to your fasting plan to ensure your well-being.

Understand Your Body's Signals

Take note of how you feel throughout the day, especially in terms of energy levels, hunger patterns, and digestion. Understanding these signals will help you select a fasting method that works with your natural rhythms rather than against them. For example, if you're typically not hungry in the morning, starting with the 16/8 method and skipping breakfast might feel natural.

Evaluate Your Nutritional Needs

Women over 60 have specific nutritional requirements, including adequate intake of calcium, vitamin D, protein, and fiber to support bone health, muscle maintenance, and digestion. Consider how fasting might affect your ability to meet these needs and plan your meals accordingly. For instance, during your eating windows, focus on nutrient-dense foods that provide the vitamins and minerals your body requires.

Consider Your Activity Level

Your level of physical activity plays a significant role in how your body responds to fasting. If you're very active, you may need a fasting method that allows for sufficient energy intake before or after exercise. For those with a more sedentary lifestyle, a longer fasting window may be easier to implement. Tailoring fasting to your activity level ensures that you maintain energy and support recovery.

Identify Any Potential Red Flags

Be mindful of any warning signs that may indicate fasting might not be suitable for you, at least without adjustments. These include:

- History of eating disorders or disordered eating habits.
- Medication schedules that require food intake.
- Sensitivity to low blood sugar or frequent dizziness.

If any of these apply to you, discuss them with a healthcare provider and consider a more moderate fasting approach, such as the 12/12 method or the 5:2 plan.

Set Realistic Goals

Finally, think about what you want to achieve with fasting. Are you looking to manage weight, improve energy, support metabolic health, or enhance overall vitality? Your goals will help guide the choice of fasting method and provide a framework for tracking your progress.

By assessing your health and understanding your body's unique needs, you can create a personalized fasting plan that is safe, effective, and sustainable. This thoughtful approach ensures that intermittent fasting becomes a supportive tool in your journey to better health, rather than a one-size-fits-all solution.

Useful Tools for Tracking Progress

Monitoring your progress is an essential part of personalizing and succeeding with intermittent fasting. By using tools to track your habits, results, and overall well-being, you can identify what works best for your body and make adjustments as needed. From apps to journals, there are a variety of tools to help you stay motivated and on track.

Fasting and Health Tracking Apps

Technology offers a convenient way to monitor your fasting schedule and progress. Many apps are specifically designed for intermittent fasting and provide features such as:

- **Fasting Timers**: Easily track the start and end of your fasting and eating windows.
- **Progress Monitoring**: Log weight, body measurements, and other metrics to see how fasting is affecting your health over time.
- **Reminders and Notifications**: Receive alerts to begin or end your fast, ensuring you stay consistent.
- **Insights and Tips**: Many apps include educational resources and personalized insights to help you optimize your fasting routine.

Popular fasting apps include **Zero**, **Fastient**, and **BodyFast**, which are user-friendly and provide customizable features to suit your needs.

Journaling

A simple journal can be one of the most effective tools for tracking your fasting journey. Writing down your daily experiences helps you stay mindful of your habits and provides valuable insights into your progress. Consider including the following in your journal:

- Your fasting and eating schedules.
- How you feel during fasting periods (e.g., energy levels, hunger, mood).
- Meals you consume during eating windows, including portion sizes and ingredients.
- Changes in physical health, such as weight, digestion, or skin clarity.
- Emotional reflections and any challenges you face.

Journaling helps you identify patterns, such as which fasting methods work best for you or which foods leave you feeling energized. Over time, it becomes a personal record of your growth and success.

Wearable Devices

If you prefer a more data-driven approach, wearable devices such as fitness trackers or smartwatches can provide detailed information about your health and activity levels. These devices can monitor:

- **Heart rate**: Fasting often lowers resting heart rate, a sign of improved cardiovascular health.
- **Sleep patterns**: Fasting can affect the quality and duration of your sleep, so tracking it can help you optimize your eating windows.
- **Physical activity**: Track steps, exercise, and calories burned to ensure you're maintaining an active lifestyle.

Brands like Fitbit, Garmin, and Apple Watch offer reliable devices that integrate with fasting apps for a seamless experience.

Photo Progress Logs

Sometimes, visual progress can be more motivating than numbers on a scale. Taking weekly or monthly photos can help you see changes in body composition, posture, and overall vitality that you might not notice otherwise.

Measurements Over Weight Alone

While many people focus on weight as a key metric, body measurements, such as waist circumference, hip size, and muscle tone, are often more accurate indicators of progress. Intermittent fasting supports fat loss while preserving muscle, so keeping track of measurements ensures you're capturing the full picture of your success.

Combining Tools for Maximum Effect

You don't have to choose just one method of tracking. Many people find that combining tools, such as using an app alongside a journal, provides a more comprehensive view of their progress. For instance, you might use an app to track fasting hours and a journal to reflect on how you feel emotionally and physically.

Tracking your progress not only keeps you accountable but also helps you celebrate small victories along the way. With the right tools, you can make intermittent fasting a sustainable and rewarding part of your lifestyle.

Guidelines for Getting Started

Start with Small Changes

When beginning your intermittent fasting journey, making small, manageable adjustments is the best way to set yourself up for success. Jumping into a strict fasting routine too quickly can feel overwhelming, but gradual changes help your body adapt naturally while building your confidence and momentum.

Choose a Method That Feels Doable

Start with a fasting schedule that aligns with your current lifestyle. For example, instead of diving into a 16/8 method, consider starting with a 12/12 approach. This means fasting for 12 hours (including sleep) and eating within a 12-hour window. As you get comfortable, you can extend your fasting period by an hour or two until you reach your desired method.

Adjust Your Meal Timing Gradually

Rather than skipping meals outright, try gradually shifting the timing of your meals. For instance, if you normally eat breakfast at 8:00 AM, delay it by 30 minutes every few days until you reach your target fasting window. Similarly, you can start having dinner slightly earlier to create a longer fasting period overnight.

Focus on Hydration

One of the simplest ways to ease into fasting is to prioritize hydration. Drinking plenty of water or herbal teas during fasting periods can help curb hunger and keep you energized. Staying hydrated also supports digestion and overall health, making the transition to fasting smoother.

Keep Your Meals Balanced

During your eating windows, focus on meals rich in nutrients, including lean proteins, healthy fats, and fiber. Avoid processed foods and refined sugars, which can cause blood sugar spikes and leave you feeling hungrier during fasting periods. Eating well-balanced meals ensures that your body gets the nutrients it needs to sustain energy and maintain muscle mass.

Start with Fewer Fasting Days

If fasting every day feels like too much, begin by practicing intermittent fasting just a few days per week. For example, you might start with fasting on Monday, Wednesday, and Friday while keeping the other days as normal eating days. This flexibility allows you to ease into fasting without feeling pressured or restricted.

Prepare Mentally and Emotionally

Before starting, set clear goals for why you want to fast. Whether it's improving energy, managing weight, or enhancing your overall health, having a clear purpose will keep you motivated. Remind yourself that it's okay to have ups and downs as you adjust to a new routine.

Be Patient with Yourself

Your body may take some time to adapt to intermittent fasting. It's normal to experience minor challenges, such as hunger or fatigue, in the beginning. These typically subside as your body becomes accustomed to fasting. Celebrate small milestones and focus on progress, not perfection.

By starting with small changes, you create a foundation for long-term success. These initial adjustments help you ease into the practice of intermittent fasting and build the confidence needed to make it a sustainable and enjoyable part of your lifestyle.

What to Do in the First Week

The first week of intermittent fasting is a crucial time for setting yourself up for long-term success. It's about building a routine, listening to your body, and easing into the practice without overwhelming yourself. Here's how to approach your first seven days with confidence and clarity.

Day 1: Start Simple

Choose a fasting method that feels manageable, such as the 12/12 approach. This means fasting for 12 hours (including sleep) and eating within a 12-hour window. For example, you might finish dinner at 7:00 PM and have breakfast at 7:00 AM the next day. Focus on getting comfortable with this schedule before extending your fasting window.

Day 2–3: Focus on Hydration

During the first few days, prioritize drinking plenty of water, herbal teas, or black coffee during fasting periods. Staying hydrated helps reduce hunger and supports your body's natural detox processes. If you feel hungry, remind yourself that this is temporary and often comes in waves.

Day 4–5: Adjust Your Meals

Pay attention to what you eat during your eating windows. Focus on nutrient-dense, whole foods that provide energy and keep you feeling full. Include lean proteins, healthy fats, and fiber-rich vegetables. Avoid processed snacks and sugary foods, which can cause energy crashes and make fasting more challenging.

Day 6: Extend Your Fasting Window (If Ready)

If you feel comfortable after five days, consider extending your fasting window by an hour or two. For example, transition from a 12/12 schedule to a 14/10 schedule, where you fast for 14 hours and eat within a 10-hour window. This gradual approach allows your body to adapt without feeling overly restricted.

Day 7: Reflect and Adjust

At the end of your first week, take time to reflect on your experience. How did your body feel during fasting periods? Were there specific times of day when hunger was more challenging? Use these insights to fine-tune your schedule and make adjustments that suit your lifestyle.

General Tips for the First Week

- **Listen to Your Body**: Pay attention to signals like energy levels, mood, and hunger. If fasting feels too difficult, consider shortening your fasting window and gradually building up.
- **Stay Busy**: Keep your mind occupied during fasting periods with activities like walking, reading, or hobbies. Distraction can help ease hunger.
- **Be Patient**: It's normal to experience minor challenges like hunger or fatigue during the first week. These typically subside as your body adjusts to fasting.
- **Celebrate Small Wins**: Completing your first fasting day or successfully extending your window is a milestone worth celebrating. Small successes build confidence and motivation.

Your first week of intermittent fasting is about experimentation and self-discovery. By focusing on progress, not perfection, you can establish a foundation for a sustainable and enjoyable fasting routine. Each day gets easier as your body adapts, bringing you closer to your health and wellness goals.

Chapter Four

Smart Nutrition During Fasting

What to Eat When Not Fasting

Essential Nutrients for Women Over 60

During eating periods, it's vital to focus on nutrient-dense foods that support your body's unique needs as you age. For women over 60, prioritizing specific nutrients helps maintain energy, preserve muscle mass, and promote overall health, ensuring that intermittent fasting works in harmony with your body.

Protein for Muscle Maintenance and Strength

Muscle mass naturally declines with age, making protein a crucial part of your diet. Adequate protein intake helps preserve and rebuild muscle, supports metabolism, and keeps you feeling full and satisfied. Include lean protein sources such as:

- Chicken, turkey, and fish.
- Eggs and low-fat dairy products like Greek yogurt or cottage cheese.
- Plant-based options such as lentils, beans, tofu, and quinoa.

Aim to include a source of protein in every meal to meet your daily requirements.

Calcium and Vitamin D for Bone Health

Bone density decreases as you age, increasing the risk of osteoporosis and fractures. Calcium and vitamin D are essential for maintaining strong, healthy bones. Incorporate calcium-rich foods like:

- Leafy greens such as kale, spinach, and broccoli.
- Dairy products like milk, cheese, and yogurt.
- Fortified plant-based milks (almond, soy, or oat).

For vitamin D, consider fatty fish like salmon or sardines, and consult your doctor about supplements if necessary.

Fiber for Digestive Health

A healthy digestive system is key to feeling your best during fasting. Fiber helps regulate bowel movements, supports gut health, and aids in managing cholesterol and blood sugar levels. Great sources of fiber include:

- Whole grains such as oats, brown rice, and whole wheat bread.
- Fruits like apples, berries, and pears.
- Vegetables such as carrots, artichokes, and Brussels sprouts.
- Legumes, nuts, and seeds.

Healthy Fats for Heart and Brain Health

Healthy fats are essential for supporting brain function, reducing inflammation, and maintaining heart health. Include sources of unsaturated fats like:

- Avocados and olive oil.

- Nuts and seeds, such as almonds, walnuts, and flaxseeds.
- Fatty fish like mackerel, trout, and salmon.

These fats not only provide energy but also help your body absorb fat-soluble vitamins like A, D, E, and K.

Antioxidants for Cellular Health

Antioxidants help combat oxidative stress, which can contribute to aging and chronic disease. Foods rich in antioxidants include:

- Brightly colored fruits and vegetables, such as blueberries, oranges, and bell peppers.
- Green tea and herbal teas.
- Spices like turmeric and cinnamon.

Hydration for Vitality

Staying hydrated is crucial for overall health, especially as dehydration becomes more common with age. Aim to drink plenty of water throughout the day, and include hydrating foods such as cucumbers, watermelon, and celery. Herbal teas and broths are also excellent choices.

Creating Balanced Meals

To maximize the benefits of intermittent fasting, aim to create balanced meals that include:

- A lean protein source.
- Healthy fats.
- Fiber-rich carbohydrates from whole grains, fruits, or vegetables.

This combination ensures you meet your body's nutritional needs while feeling full and energized during your eating windows.

By prioritizing these essential nutrients, you can make the most of your eating periods, support your body's unique needs, and complement the benefits of fasting for a healthier, more vibrant life.

Examples of Healthy and Balanced Meals

Eating balanced, nutrient-dense meals during your eating window is essential for complementing the benefits of intermittent fasting. A well-rounded meal provides the energy, vitamins, and minerals your body needs to thrive while keeping you satisfied and supporting overall health. Below are examples of balanced meals tailored for women over 60, emphasizing essential nutrients like protein, fiber, healthy fats, and antioxidants.

Breakfast Options

1. **Greek Yogurt Bowl with Berries and Nuts**
   - **Ingredients:** 1 cup of plain Greek yogurt (high in protein and calcium), ½ cup of mixed berries (rich in antioxidants), 1 tablespoon of chia seeds (fiber and omega-3s), and a handful of almonds or walnuts (healthy fats).
   - **Benefits:** Supports digestion, provides long-lasting energy, and is easy to prepare.

2. **Vegetable Omelet with Whole Grain Toast**
   - **Ingredients:** 2 eggs (protein and essential nutrients), sautéed spinach, mushrooms, and bell peppers (fiber and vitamins), and a slice of whole-grain toast.
   - **Benefits:** High in protein and fiber to keep you full and energized, with healthy fats from the eggs.

3. **Overnight Oats with Fruit and Nut Butter**
   - **Ingredients:** ½ cup of rolled oats, 1 cup of unsweetened almond milk, 1 tablespoon of almond butter, ½ banana (potassium), and a sprinkle of cinnamon (anti-inflammatory).

- **Benefits:** A fiber-packed, easy-to-digest meal that supports heart health and stable energy levels.

Lunch Options

1. **Grilled Chicken Salad with Avocado and Olive Oil Dressing**
   - **Ingredients:** Mixed greens (romaine, spinach, arugula), grilled chicken breast (lean protein), ½ avocado (healthy fats), cherry tomatoes, cucumbers, and a dressing made with extra virgin olive oil and lemon juice.
   - **Benefits:** High in protein and fiber, with heart-healthy fats and antioxidants.

2. **Quinoa Bowl with Roasted Vegetables and Chickpeas**
   - **Ingredients**: 1 cup of cooked quinoa (a complete plant-based protein), roasted sweet potatoes and Brussels sprouts (fiber and vitamins), ½ cup of chickpeas, and a drizzle of tahini.
   - **Benefits**: A filling, plant-based option rich in protein and nutrients for sustained energy.

3. **Turkey and Avocado Wrap with a Side Salad**
   - **Ingredients**: A whole-grain wrap, sliced turkey breast (lean protein), ½ avocado, lettuce, tomato, and mustard, served with a side of mixed greens.
   - **Benefits**: Balanced with protein, fiber, and healthy fats to keep you satisfied.

Dinner Options

1. **Grilled Salmon with Steamed Broccoli and Brown Rice**
   - Ingredients: 4 oz of salmon (omega-3 fatty acids), 1 cup of steamed broccoli (fiber and antioxidants), and ½ cup of cooked brown rice (complex carbohydrates).

- Benefits: Supports brain health and heart health while providing sustained energy.

2. **Lean Beef Stir-Fry with Vegetables and Quinoa**

- **Ingredients:** 4 oz of lean beef strips, a mix of stir-fried vegetables (like bell peppers, snap peas, and carrots), and 1 cup of cooked quinoa. Use a low-sodium soy sauce for flavor.
- **Benefits:** High in protein, fiber, and essential nutrients to support muscle health and digestion.

3. **Baked Cod with Sweet Potato Mash and Asparagus**

- **Ingredients:** 4 oz of cod (low-fat protein), 1 medium sweet potato mashed with a touch of olive oil, and roasted asparagus (rich in vitamins and minerals).
- **Benefits:** Provides a balance of lean protein, healthy carbs, and fiber.

Snacks and Small Meals

For smaller meals or snacks within your eating window, consider these nutrient-dense options:

- A handful of mixed nuts and a piece of fruit, such as an apple or pear.
- Cottage cheese with sliced cucumbers and a sprinkle of black pepper.
- A boiled egg with a small avocado.
- Hummus with carrot and celery sticks.

Key Tips for Balanced Meals

- **Include all macronutrients**: Each meal should have a source of protein, healthy fats, and fiber-rich carbohydrates to keep you full and energized.
- **Focus on whole foods**: Avoid processed and sugary foods that can cause energy crashes.

- **Add variety**: Rotate your meals to include a wide range of nutrients and keep your diet enjoyable.
- **Hydrate**: Drink water or herbal tea with meals to support digestion and hydration.

These balanced meal examples are designed to support your body's needs while complementing your intermittent fasting schedule. With a little planning, you can create delicious, satisfying meals that enhance your health and vitality.

Foods That Enhance Fasting

Superfoods for Energy and Longevity

Incorporating superfoods into your diet during eating periods can amplify the benefits of intermittent fasting. These nutrient-dense foods provide essential vitamins, minerals, antioxidants, and healthy fats that support energy, cellular repair, and overall longevity. For women over 60, these foods are especially valuable in promoting vitality and addressing age-related health concerns.

1. Leafy Greens

Dark, leafy greens like spinach, kale, and Swiss chard are packed with vitamins A, C, and K, along with minerals like calcium and magnesium. They support bone health, reduce inflammation, and provide antioxidants to combat oxidative stress. Adding these greens to salads, smoothies, or cooked meals can boost your nutrient intake significantly.

2. Fatty Fish

Salmon, mackerel, and sardines are excellent sources of omega-3 fatty acids, which are crucial for brain health, heart health, and reducing inflammation. Omega-3s also help regulate hormones, making them particularly beneficial for women post-menopause. Including fatty fish in your diet two to three times per week is ideal for longevity and energy.

3. Berries

Blueberries, strawberries, raspberries, and blackberries are rich in antioxidants and low in calories, making them perfect for supporting fasting. Their high levels of anthocyanins help protect cells from damage, improve brain function, and support cardiovascular health. They also provide natural sweetness without spiking blood sugar levels.

4. Nuts and Seeds

Almonds, walnuts, chia seeds, and flaxseeds are excellent sources of healthy fats, protein, and fiber. They keep you feeling full longer and provide essential nutrients like magnesium, zinc, and omega-3 fatty acids. Sprinkle them over yogurt, salads, or oatmeal for an easy nutritional boost.

5. Avocados

Avocados are a powerhouse of healthy monounsaturated fats, potassium, and fiber. They promote heart health, support digestion, and provide lasting energy. Avocados can be enjoyed as a spread, in salads, or simply sliced as a side to your main meal.

6. Turmeric

This golden spice contains curcumin, a powerful anti-inflammatory and antioxidant compound. Turmeric supports joint health, brain function, and immune response. Adding a pinch of turmeric to soups, teas, or roasted vegetables can enhance your meals and your health.

7. Green Tea

Green tea is a fasting-friendly drink that provides a gentle caffeine boost and is rich in catechins, which help with fat oxidation and reduce inflammation. Drinking green tea during fasting periods can enhance fat burning, while during eating windows, it supports overall metabolic health.

8. Sweet Potatoes

Sweet potatoes are an excellent source of complex carbohydrates, beta-carotene, and fiber. They provide sustained energy without spiking blood sugar levels, making them an ideal addition to your eating periods. Enjoy them roasted, mashed, or added to soups and stews.

9. Fermented Foods

Foods like yogurt, kefir, sauerkraut, and kimchi are rich in probiotics, which support gut health and digestion. A healthy gut microbiome is essential for nutrient absorption and overall well-being, especially as digestion can slow with age.

10. Dark Chocolate

Dark chocolate with a cocoa content of 70% or higher is packed with antioxidants and flavonoids that support heart health and brain function. Enjoying a small square during your eating window can be a satisfying and healthful treat.

How to Incorporate These Superfoods

- **Make them a staple**: Include at least one or two superfoods in each meal to ensure you're meeting your nutritional needs.
- **Combine flavors**: Pair superfoods for even greater benefits, such as a salad with spinach, avocado, and nuts, or a smoothie with berries, flaxseeds, and yogurt.

- **Keep it simple**: Superfoods are versatile and easy to prepare, making them accessible even on busy days.

By incorporating these superfoods into your diet, you can maximize the energy-boosting and longevity-promoting benefits of intermittent fasting. These nutrient-rich options not only nourish your body but also enhance your overall well-being, helping you thrive at every stage of life.

Foods That Stimulate Autophagy

Autophagy, the body's natural cellular "clean-up" process, is a key benefit of intermittent fasting. This process removes damaged cells, recycles their components, and promotes the generation of new, healthy cells. While fasting is a primary trigger for autophagy, certain foods can enhance and support this process during your eating periods. Incorporating these foods into your diet helps optimize the benefits of autophagy, supporting longevity, reduced inflammation, and overall cellular health.

1. Green Tea

Rich in compounds like catechins and polyphenols, green tea has been shown to enhance autophagy, particularly in the brain. Drinking green tea during or after your fasting period can support cellular repair and protect against neurodegenerative diseases. Matcha, a powdered form of green tea, offers an even more concentrated source of these beneficial compounds.

2. Turmeric

Curcumin, the active ingredient in turmeric, is a powerful anti-inflammatory agent that also stimulates autophagy. Turmeric can be added to meals, soups, or teas, making it an easy and flavorful addition to your diet.

For better absorption, pair turmeric with black pepper, which enhances curcumin's bioavailability.

3. Cruciferous Vegetables

Broccoli, cauliflower, Brussels sprouts, and kale contain sulforaphane, a compound known to promote autophagy and protect against cellular damage. These vegetables are also high in fiber and antioxidants, which support digestion and overall health.

4. Extra Virgin Olive Oil

A staple of the Mediterranean diet, extra virgin olive oil contains healthy fats and polyphenols that stimulate autophagy and combat oxidative stress. Drizzle olive oil over salads, roasted vegetables, or whole-grain bread to enjoy its benefits.

5. Garlic

Garlic is rich in sulfur compounds that support detoxification and stimulate autophagy, particularly in the liver. Adding fresh garlic to your cooking not only enhances flavor but also boosts your body's ability to repair and regenerate cells.

6. Nuts and Seeds

Walnuts, almonds, flaxseeds, and chia seeds are rich in omega-3 fatty acids and polyphenols, which enhance autophagy and reduce inflammation. These nutrient-dense foods are also excellent sources of energy during your eating window.

7. Berries

Blueberries, blackberries, and raspberries are packed with anthocyanins, antioxidants that trigger autophagy and protect cells from oxidative damage. These fruits also support brain health and reduce inflammation, making them a valuable addition to your diet.

8. Seaweed

Rich in iodine, antioxidants, and unique bioactive compounds, seaweed promotes autophagy and supports thyroid health. Add seaweed to soups, salads, or enjoy it as a snack in dried form.

9. Apple Cider Vinegar

This fermented tonic has been linked to improved insulin sensitivity and autophagy activation. A tablespoon of apple cider vinegar diluted in water before meals can help enhance digestion and support cellular health.

10. Dark Chocolate

Dark chocolate with a high cocoa content (70% or more) contains flavonoids that activate autophagy and reduce inflammation. Enjoying a small piece during your eating window can be both satisfying and health-promoting.

Incorporating These Foods into Your Diet

To maximize the autophagy-boosting benefits of these foods:

- Include a variety of them in your meals to ensure a broad spectrum of nutrients.
- Pair autophagy-friendly foods with intermittent fasting to create a synergistic effect. For example, break your fast with a meal that includes broccoli, olive oil, and garlic.
- Use simple recipes that highlight these foods without heavy processing or added sugars, which can counteract their benefits.

By intentionally adding these autophagy-promoting foods to your diet, you can enhance your body's natural repair processes and unlock greater health and vitality. Combined with fasting, these foods create a powerful strategy for supporting long-term cellular health and longevity.

What to Avoid

Foods That Can Sabotage Fasting

While intermittent fasting allows flexibility in what you eat during your eating windows, certain foods can undermine its benefits. These foods may disrupt metabolic processes, hinder fat burning, and even make fasting periods more challenging by causing hunger spikes or energy crashes. Being mindful of what you consume ensures that your fasting efforts are effective and sustainable.

1. Sugary Foods and Drinks

Consuming foods and beverages high in added sugar, such as candies, pastries, sugary cereals, and soda, can cause rapid spikes in blood sugar followed by sharp crashes. These fluctuations lead to increased hunger, irritability, and difficulty maintaining energy levels during fasting periods. Instead, opt for naturally sweet foods like fruits, which provide fiber and nutrients without destabilizing blood sugar.

2. Refined Carbohydrates

White bread, white rice, pasta, and other refined grains are quickly broken down into glucose, leading to similar blood sugar spikes and crashes. These foods offer little nutritional value and can leave you feeling hungrier sooner. Choose whole grains like quinoa, brown rice, or whole-grain bread, which provide sustained energy and essential nutrients.

3. Fried and Processed Foods

Foods like fried chicken, French fries, and processed snacks are high in unhealthy trans fats and empty calories. These foods can lead to inflammation, weight gain, and sluggish digestion, counteracting the benefits of fasting. Instead, prepare meals with healthy cooking methods like grilling, steaming, or roasting.

4. Highly Processed Snacks

Chips, crackers, and other packaged snacks often contain high levels of sodium, unhealthy fats, and artificial additives. These ingredients can increase water retention, lead to bloating, and provide little satiety. Replace these with nutrient-dense snacks like nuts, seeds, or fresh veggies.

5. Alcohol

Alcoholic beverages disrupt the body's natural detoxification processes, increase dehydration, and add empty calories with no nutritional value. Drinking alcohol during your eating windows can also interfere with the restorative processes activated by fasting. If you choose to drink, limit it to small amounts and opt for lower-sugar options like dry wine.

6. Artificial Sweeteners

While calorie-free, artificial sweeteners in diet sodas, sugar-free desserts, and other products can disrupt gut health and increase sugar cravings. They may also trigger insulin responses, which can undermine the metabolic benefits of fasting. If you need a sweetener, opt for natural alternatives like stevia or monk fruit in moderation.

7. Large, Heavy Meals

Eating oversized portions or meals high in unhealthy fats can make digestion sluggish and leave you feeling uncomfortable, especially if you're breaking your fast. Focus on smaller, balanced meals that are easy to digest and rich in nutrients to optimize energy levels.

8. Packaged and Pre-Made Foods

Many pre-made meals, frozen dinners, and canned soups are loaded with preservatives, sodium, and unhealthy fats. These additives can contribute to bloating and inflammation, counteracting fasting's health benefits. Preparing fresh, homemade meals gives you better control over the quality of your food.

9. Excessive Caffeine

While moderate amounts of black coffee or tea can enhance fasting, overconsuming caffeine can lead to dehydration, jitters, and digestive discomfort. Be mindful of your intake and balance caffeinated drinks with water or herbal teas.

10. Low-Fat or "Diet" Foods

Many "diet" or "low-fat" products are highly processed and contain added sugars or artificial ingredients to compensate for reduced fat content. These foods can cause hunger spikes and cravings, making fasting more difficult. Stick to whole, unprocessed foods for a more satisfying and nutritious diet.

Key Tips for Success

- Prioritize whole, unprocessed foods that nourish your body and keep you full longer.
- Focus on meals rich in protein, fiber, and healthy fats to maintain stable blood sugar levels.
- Avoid foods that leave you feeling bloated, fatigued, or excessively hungry, as they can make fasting less enjoyable.

By steering clear of these foods, you can enhance the benefits of intermittent fasting and make your fasting periods more manageable. Choosing nourishing, high-quality ingredients will help you feel energized, satisfied, and ready to embrace your fasting journey with confidence.

Common Mistakes to Avoid

Intermittent fasting can be a highly effective and sustainable practice, but certain mistakes can hinder your progress or make the experience more challenging than necessary. Being aware of these common pitfalls ensures you maximize the benefits of fasting while maintaining a balanced and enjoyable lifestyle.

1. Overeating During Eating Windows

One of the most frequent mistakes is consuming excessive amounts of food during eating periods. While it's natural to feel hungry after fasting, overeating can lead to bloating, sluggishness, and weight gain. Focus on balanced meals that include protein, fiber, and healthy fats to keep you satisfied without overloading your system.

2. Choosing Unhealthy Foods

Another common error is indulging in processed, sugary, or fried foods during eating windows. These choices can cause energy crashes, disrupt blood sugar levels, and counteract the benefits of fasting. Prioritize whole, nutrient-dense foods that provide lasting energy and support overall health.

3. Not Drinking Enough Water

Dehydration is a common issue during fasting periods. Many people mistake thirst for hunger, which can make fasting more difficult. Drink plenty of water throughout the day and consider adding herbal teas or sparkling water to stay hydrated and curb hunger.

4. Jumping Into Long Fasting Windows Too Quickly

Starting with extended fasting periods, such as 24-hour fasts or OMAD (One Meal a Day), without prior experience can feel overwhelming and lead to fatigue or irritability. Begin with shorter windows, like 12/12 or 16/8, and gradually increase the duration as your body adapts.

5. Ignoring Your Body's Signals

Fasting is not a one-size-fits-all approach. Ignoring symptoms like dizziness, extreme fatigue, or persistent hunger can be harmful. Listen to your body and make adjustments if needed, such as shortening your fasting window or choosing a more flexible method like the 5:2 approach.

6. Neglecting Nutrition

Some people focus solely on fasting and overlook the quality of their meals. Skipping essential nutrients like protein, healthy fats, and fiber can leave you feeling tired and make fasting unsustainable. Plan balanced meals to ensure you meet your body's nutritional needs.

7. Consuming Hidden Calories During Fasting

Unknowingly consuming calories during fasting periods—such as adding cream and sugar to coffee or snacking on small bites—can disrupt the fasting process. Stick to calorie-free beverages like water, black coffee, or herbal tea during fasting hours.

8. Expecting Immediate Results

Fasting is not a quick fix, and expecting dramatic weight loss or health improvements in the first few days can lead to frustration. Focusing on consistency and small, sustainable changes will yield better results over time.

9. Overexercising While Adjusting to Fasting

While staying active is important, excessive or high-intensity exercise during fasting—especially in the beginning—can leave you feeling drained. Start with light activities like walking, yoga, or stretching and gradually increase intensity as your body adapts to fasting.

10. Being Too Rigid

Being overly strict with your fasting schedule can lead to unnecessary stress. Life happens, and it's okay to adjust your plan occasionally. Flexibility is key to making intermittent fasting a long-term and enjoyable part of your lifestyle.

How to Avoid These Mistakes

- **Plan Ahead**: Prepare balanced meals and snacks in advance to avoid making poor food choices during eating windows.
- **Start Slow**: Gradually ease into fasting and increase your fasting windows over time.
- **Track Your Progress**: Use a journal or app to monitor how your body responds to fasting and make adjustments as needed.
- **Stay Flexible**: Focus on consistency rather than perfection, allowing room for adjustments when necessary.

By avoiding these common mistakes and approaching fasting with a mindful, balanced strategy, you can enjoy its many benefits while creating a routine that fits your life and supports your health goals.

Chapter Five

Fasting and an Active Lifestyle

The Importance of Physical Activity

Recommended Exercises for Women Over 60

Incorporating physical activity into your routine is essential for enhancing the benefits of intermittent fasting. For women over 60, exercise supports muscle maintenance, improves bone health, boosts energy, and enhances overall well-being. The key is to choose activities that are enjoyable, safe, and effective for your body at this stage of life. Here are some of the best types of exercises to complement your fasting lifestyle.

1. Strength Training

Maintaining muscle mass becomes increasingly important as we age, as it naturally declines over time. Strength training helps preserve muscle, improve metabolism, and support joint health.

- **Examples**: Bodyweight exercises like squats, lunges, and push-ups, or light resistance training with dumbbells, resistance bands, or kettlebells.
- **Frequency**: Aim for 2–3 sessions per week, targeting major muscle groups.
- **Tips**: Start with light weights and gradually increase resistance to avoid injury.

2. Walking

Walking is a low-impact, accessible exercise that improves cardiovascular health, promotes fat burning, and enhances mental clarity.

- **Examples**: Brisk walks in your neighborhood, on a treadmill, or in a park.
- **Frequency**: Aim for 30 minutes a day, 5–7 days per week.
- **Tips**: Incorporate walking into your daily routine, such as taking a stroll after meals to aid digestion and stabilize blood sugar.

3. Yoga

Yoga is excellent for improving flexibility, balance, and strength while reducing stress. It's particularly beneficial for women over 60, as it supports joint mobility and prevents stiffness.

- **Examples**: Gentle yoga or restorative yoga classes, or poses like downward dog, cat-cow, and warrior poses.
- **Frequency**: Practice 2–4 times per week.
- **Tips**: Look for classes or online tutorials designed for beginners or seniors.

4. Pilates

Pilates focuses on core strength, posture, and flexibility, making it a great option for enhancing mobility and preventing injuries.

- **Examples**: Mat Pilates or exercises using a stability ball or reformer.

- **Frequency**: 1–3 sessions per week.
- **Tips**: Start with beginner classes to learn proper form and technique.

5. Swimming and Water Aerobics

Water-based exercises are gentle on the joints while providing a full-body workout. They're particularly useful for women with arthritis or joint pain.

- **Examples**: Swimming laps, water aerobics classes, or simply walking in a pool.
- **Frequency**: 2–3 times per week.
- **Tips**: Look for heated pools if you have arthritis, as warm water can soothe joints and muscles.

6. Stretching and Mobility Exercises

Stretching helps improve flexibility, reduce muscle tension, and maintain range of motion. Mobility exercises ensure joints remain functional and healthy.

- **Examples**: Dynamic stretches, foam rolling, or gentle movements like arm circles and hip openers.
- **Frequency**: Incorporate stretching into your daily routine, particularly after workouts or fasting periods.

7. Low-Impact Cardio

Cardiovascular exercise supports heart health and increases endurance without straining the joints.

- **Examples**: Cycling, elliptical training, or dancing.
- **Frequency**: 3–5 sessions per week, lasting 20–40 minutes each.
- **Tips**: Focus on moderate intensity to avoid overexertion.

Creating a Balanced Routine

- **Mix Activities**: Combine strength training, cardio, and flexibility exercises for a well-rounded routine.
- **Adjust for Fasting**: Plan workouts during your eating window or when you feel most energized. Light activities like yoga or walking are great for fasting periods.
- **Listen to Your Body**: Modify exercises as needed to suit your fitness level and avoid pushing through pain.

By incorporating these recommended exercises into your routine, you can amplify the benefits of fasting, improve your overall health, and enjoy a more active, fulfilling lifestyle. Fitness at any age is about finding what works for you and staying consistent—your body and mind will thank you for it!

Light Workouts: Yoga, Stretching, and Walking

For women over 60, light workouts such as yoga, stretching, and walking offer a gentle yet effective way to stay active and complement the benefits of intermittent fasting. These activities are easy on the joints, improve mobility, and provide mental clarity, making them an excellent choice for maintaining a healthy, active lifestyle.

Yoga

Yoga is a versatile practice that enhances flexibility, balance, and strength while reducing stress and promoting mindfulness. It's particularly beneficial for women over 60 as it supports joint health and helps alleviate stiffness.

- **Benefits**: Improves posture, reduces tension, and enhances circulation. Yoga also helps calm the mind, which is especially helpful during fasting periods.
- **Recommended Poses**:
  o *Cat-Cow*: To improve spine flexibility.
  o *Child's Pose*: For gentle stretching of the back and hips.
  o *Warrior II*: To build strength and stability.
- **Tips**: Start with beginner or restorative yoga classes, either in-person or online. Use props like blocks and straps for added support and comfort.

Stretching

Stretching is essential for maintaining range of motion and preventing injuries. It's especially important for women over 60 to combat the natural loss of flexibility that comes with aging.

- **Benefits**: Reduces muscle tension, improves joint mobility, and supports better posture. Stretching also aids in recovery after workouts and fasting periods.
- **Examples of Stretches**:
  o *Hamstring Stretch*: Sit on the floor with one leg extended and reach for your toes.
  o *Shoulder Rolls*: To release tension in the shoulders and neck.
  o *Seated Spinal Twist*: To improve spinal mobility.
- **Tips**: Hold each stretch for 20–30 seconds and avoid bouncing. Stretch daily, especially after light activity or long periods of sitting.

Walking

Walking is one of the simplest and most accessible forms of exercise. It's low-impact, easy to incorporate into daily life, and highly effective for improving cardiovascular health and boosting mood.

- **Benefits**: Promotes fat burning, supports joint health, and enhances mental clarity. Walking also aids digestion and stabilizes blood sugar levels when done after meals.
- **How to Get Started**:
  o Begin with 10–15-minute walks and gradually increase to 30–45 minutes daily.
  o Walk at a pace that feels comfortable but slightly challenging.
  o Choose scenic routes or walk with a friend to make it enjoyable.
- **Tips**: Wear supportive shoes to protect your joints and try to include hills or varied terrain for added benefits.

How to Incorporate Light Workouts into Your Routine

- **Daily Practice**: Dedicate 10–20 minutes each day to yoga or stretching, and aim for a 30-minute walk at least five days a week.
- **Combine Activities**: For example, start with a short walk, followed by a gentle yoga session or targeted stretching.
- **Adjust for Fasting**: These light workouts are ideal during fasting periods when energy levels may be lower, as they don't require intense exertion.

By incorporating yoga, stretching, and walking into your lifestyle, you can enjoy improved flexibility, reduced stress, and enhanced overall well-being. These gentle activities are perfect for supporting your body during fasting and ensuring you stay active and energized as you age.

Managing Stress and Sleep

How Fasting Improves Sleep

Intermittent fasting can have a positive impact on sleep quality by promoting natural rhythms in the body, improving metabolic health, and reducing factors that disrupt rest. For women over 60, better sleep means improved energy, mental clarity, and overall well-being. Here's how fasting supports a more restful night's sleep.

1. Regulates Circadian Rhythms

Intermittent fasting aligns eating patterns with the body's natural circadian rhythms, the 24-hour internal clock that regulates sleep-wake cycles. Eating during daylight hours and fasting at night helps the body maintain a consistent rhythm, promoting better sleep. Fasting reduces late-night eating, which can interfere with the release of melatonin, the hormone that signals your body it's time to rest.

2. Improves Digestion for Better Rest

Eating late in the evening can cause indigestion or discomfort that disrupts sleep. By fasting for several hours before bedtime, your digestive system has time to rest, reducing the likelihood of issues like acid reflux or bloating. This allows your body to fully focus on restorative processes during sleep, rather than digesting food.

3. Stabilizes Blood Sugar Levels

Blood sugar fluctuations, particularly at night, can wake you up or prevent deep, restorative sleep. Intermittent fasting helps regulate insulin sensitivity and stabilize blood sugar levels, reducing nighttime energy crashes or spikes that might interrupt sleep.

4. Reduces Stress and Cortisol Levels

Fasting has been shown to lower cortisol, the stress hormone that, when elevated, can disrupt sleep patterns. A well-implemented fasting routine reduces stress on the body, creating a calmer state that promotes relaxation and makes it easier to fall asleep and stay asleep.

5. Enhances Production of Growth Hormones

During fasting, the body naturally increases the production of human growth hormone (HGH). HGH supports cell repair, tissue growth, and overall recovery, processes that are most active during deep sleep. This enhanced repair cycle improves the quality of rest and leaves you feeling more refreshed in the morning.

6. Encourages a Balanced Lifestyle

By promoting mindful eating and reducing late-night snacking, fasting encourages a more structured routine that prioritizes rest and recovery. This balanced approach not only improves sleep but also creates a healthier, more sustainable lifestyle overall.

Tips for Combining Fasting and Sleep

- **Finish Eating Early**: Aim to stop eating at least 3–4 hours before bedtime to allow your body to wind down and prepare for sleep.
- **Avoid Stimulants**: Limit caffeine and sugar during your eating window, especially in the afternoon and evening, to prevent sleep disruptions.
- **Stick to a Schedule**: Consistent eating and fasting windows help regulate your circadian rhythm, supporting regular sleep patterns.

By improving metabolic health, reducing nighttime disruptions, and aligning with natural rhythms, intermittent fasting supports better sleep quality. For women over 60, this means waking up feeling rejuvenated and ready to embrace the day with energy and focus.

Relaxation Techniques: Meditation and Mindfulness

Incorporating relaxation techniques like meditation and mindfulness into your routine can greatly enhance the benefits of intermittent fasting. These practices reduce stress, improve mental clarity, and promote emotional balance, making it easier to maintain a healthy and active lifestyle. For women over 60, meditation and mindfulness can be transformative tools for managing the natural challenges of aging and fasting.

The Benefits of Meditation and Mindfulness

Meditation and mindfulness are practices that help you focus on the present moment, reducing stress and improving overall well-being. They are particularly beneficial during fasting periods when stress or hunger might arise. Benefits include:

- **Lower stress levels**: By calming the mind, these techniques reduce cortisol, the stress hormone, which can interfere with fasting and overall health.
- **Improved focus and clarity**: A clear mind helps you stay committed to your fasting goals and navigate challenges.
- **Enhanced emotional resilience**: Mindfulness helps you recognize and respond to emotions, such as hunger or frustration, in a calm and constructive way.

- **Better sleep**: Relaxation techniques prepare your mind and body for restful sleep by reducing tension and promoting relaxation.

Meditation Techniques

1. **Guided Meditation**
   - Use apps or online videos to follow a guided session.
   - Focus on a calming voice or visualization to center your mind.
2. **Breath Awareness Meditation**
   - Sit comfortably, close your eyes, and focus on your breathing.
   - Inhale deeply through your nose, hold for a moment, and exhale slowly.
   - Pay attention to the sensation of air entering and leaving your body.
3. **Mantra Meditation**
   - Choose a calming word or phrase (e.g., "peace" or "I am calm").
   - Silently repeat the mantra as you breathe, letting it guide your focus.

Mindfulness Practices

1. **Mindful Eating**
   - During your eating window, pay close attention to the texture, taste, and smell of your food.
   - Chew slowly and savor each bite, which improves digestion and helps prevent overeating.
2. **Body Scan Technique**
   - Lie down or sit comfortably and close your eyes.
   - Slowly focus your attention on different parts of your body, starting from your toes and moving upward.
   - Notice any tension or discomfort and consciously relax those areas.

3. **Mindful Walking**
   o Take a slow, deliberate walk, focusing on the sensation of your feet touching the ground, the rhythm of your breathing, and the sounds around you.
   o This practice doubles as light exercise and relaxation.

Incorporating Relaxation Techniques into Your Day

- **Morning Practice**: Start your day with a 5–10 minute meditation to set a positive tone.
- **During Fasting Periods**: Use mindfulness to manage hunger waves or stress by focusing on your breathing or repeating a calming mantra.
- **Evening Wind-Down**: End your day with a body scan or guided meditation to prepare for restful sleep.

Relaxation techniques like meditation and mindfulness are simple yet powerful tools for enhancing your fasting journey. They help you stay grounded, reduce stress, and create a more harmonious connection between your mind and body. By dedicating a few moments each day to these practices, you can amplify the physical and emotional benefits of intermittent fasting and cultivate a deeper sense of well-being.

Creating a Daily Rhythm

How to Incorporate Fasting into Your Daily Routine

Integrating intermittent fasting into your daily routine is about finding a rhythm that aligns with your lifestyle, energy levels, and personal goals. For women over 60, a well-planned fasting routine not only supports physical health but also promotes balance and consistency throughout the day. Here's how to seamlessly incorporate fasting into your life.

1. Choose a Fasting Schedule That Fits Your Lifestyle

Start by selecting a fasting method that works with your daily activities and natural eating patterns. For example:

- **16/8 Method**: Fast for 16 hours (including sleep) and eat within an 8-hour window, such as 11:00 AM to 7:00 PM.
- **12/12 Method**: Fast for 12 hours and eat within the remaining 12 hours, ideal for beginners.
- **5:2 Method**: Eat normally five days a week and reduce calorie intake on two non-consecutive days.

Match your fasting window to your most convenient or least stressful hours.

2. Time Meals Around Energy Levels

Pay attention to when you feel most energetic or hungry during the day. Many women prefer breaking their fast with a mid-morning meal and finishing their eating window with an early dinner. Adjust your schedule to suit your unique rhythm.

3. Plan Meals in Advance

Planning your meals for the day ensures you stay on track and avoid unhealthy choices.

- Prepare nutrient-dense meals that include lean proteins, healthy fats, and fiber to keep you satisfied.
- Have quick, healthy snacks ready for your eating window, such as nuts, yogurt, or cut-up vegetables, to avoid grabbing processed foods.

4. Use Fasting-Friendly Beverages

During fasting periods, stay hydrated with water, herbal teas, or black coffee. These beverages help suppress hunger, maintain energy, and support your body's natural detox processes without breaking your fast.

5. Align Fasting with Daily Activities

Incorporate fasting into your existing routine:

- **Morning**: Use this time for light activities like yoga, walking, or meditation to ease into your day while fasting.
- **Afternoon**: Plan meals around lunch or early dinner to maximize your eating window.
- **Evening**: Focus on relaxation and avoid eating late to support your circadian rhythm and improve sleep.

6. Stay Flexible

Life can be unpredictable, and it's okay to adjust your fasting schedule when needed. If you have social events, holidays, or unexpected commitments, shift your fasting or eating window to accommodate your plans without stress.

7. Track Your Progress

Use a journal or app to monitor how fasting fits into your routine. Record your fasting hours, meals, energy levels, and mood to identify what works best for you and make adjustments as needed.

8. Combine Fasting with Healthy Habits

Enhance your fasting routine by incorporating complementary habits:

- **Exercise**: Schedule light to moderate workouts during your fasting period or eating window, depending on your energy levels.
- **Sleep**: Aim for 7–8 hours of restful sleep each night to support your body's recovery.

- **Stress Management**: Practice mindfulness or meditation to maintain a sense of balance and calm.

Example Daily Routine for the 16/8 Method
- **7:00 AM**: Start your day with a glass of water or herbal tea.
- **8:00 AM**: Go for a light walk or practice yoga.
- **11:00 AM**: Break your fast with a balanced meal (e.g., Greek yogurt with nuts and berries).
- **2:00 PM**: Enjoy a nutrient-dense lunch (e.g., a grilled chicken salad with avocado and olive oil).
- **6:30 PM**: Finish your eating window with a light dinner (e.g., baked salmon with steamed vegetables).
- **7:00 PM–Bedtime**: Hydrate with water or herbal tea, relax with stretching or reading, and prepare for restful sleep.

By integrating fasting into your daily routine in a way that feels natural and sustainable, you can enjoy its many benefits without disrupting your lifestyle. Consistency, preparation, and flexibility are key to making fasting a seamless and rewarding part of your day.

The Importance of Consistency

Consistency is the foundation of success in intermittent fasting. Like any new habit, fasting requires time, patience, and dedication to yield its full benefits. For women over 60, maintaining a steady routine not only enhances the effectiveness of fasting but also creates a sense of balance and control in daily life.

When you approach fasting with consistency, your body begins to adapt to the new eating and fasting schedule. Over time, hunger signals become more predictable, energy levels stabilize, and the process feels more natural. This adaptation reduces the initial challenges, such as hunger pangs or fatigue, making fasting a sustainable and enjoyable practice.

Sticking to a regular routine also strengthens the positive habits that support your overall health. By eating nutrient-dense meals during your eating windows, hydrating properly, and aligning fasting with your daily activities, you create a rhythm that promotes well-being and longevity. Consistency ensures that these habits become second nature, requiring less effort and conscious thought over time.

It's important to remember that consistency doesn't mean perfection. Life can bring unexpected challenges, such as social events, travel, or changes in schedule. What matters most is your ability to return to your fasting routine with confidence after these moments. A flexible but steady approach ensures long-term success without unnecessary stress.

By committing to a consistent practice of intermittent fasting, you give your body and mind the stability they need to thrive. This commitment not only enhances the physical benefits of fasting but also builds resilience, self-discipline, and a greater sense of empowerment in your health journey.

Chapter Six

Testimonials and Inspiration

Success Stories

Real Testimonials from Women Over 60

Hearing from women who have successfully incorporated intermittent fasting into their lives can be incredibly motivating. Their stories demonstrate that age is no barrier to achieving better health, more energy, and greater confidence. These real-life experiences showcase how intermittent fasting can transform not only the body but also the mind and spirit.

Susan, 64 – Finding Energy and Focus: Susan, a retired teacher, had struggled with fatigue and lack of focus for years. After starting the 16/8 fasting method, she noticed a remarkable difference. "I used to feel sluggish in the afternoons, but now I have energy all day. Fasting has helped me structure my meals better, and I'm amazed at how much sharper I feel. It's like I've reclaimed my vitality."

Margaret, 68 – Managing Weight and Diabetes: For Margaret, a grandmother of four, managing her type 2 diabetes was a constant challenge. After consulting with her doctor, she started intermittent fasting with the 5:2 method. "It was a bit tough at first, but I eased into it. Now, my blood sugar levels are more stable, and I've lost 15 pounds over six months. It's not just about the weight—I feel like I've taken control of my health."

Linda, 61 – Overcoming Emotional Eating: Linda, a former nurse, found herself turning to food for comfort after retiring. Intermittent fasting helped her rebuild a healthier relationship with eating. "I learned to listen to my body and eat when I'm truly hungry. Fasting has been a game-changer for me—not just physically, but emotionally. I've lost 10 pounds, and I feel more in tune with myself."

Catherine, 70 – Staying Active and Strong: Catherine, an avid gardener and yoga enthusiast, was looking for a way to stay active and maintain muscle strength as she aged. She incorporated the 16/8 fasting method into her routine and focused on nutrient-dense meals. "I love how fasting fits into my lifestyle. I've kept my energy levels high for gardening and yoga, and I feel stronger than ever. Fasting has become a part of my life, not a chore."

Barbara, 63 – Boosting Confidence and Wellness: Barbara, who works part-time in a bookstore, embraced intermittent fasting as a way to prioritize her health. "I was hesitant at first, but the simplicity of fasting won me over. I've lost inches around my waist, and my confidence has soared. Fasting has reminded me that it's never too late to invest in yourself."

The Common Thread

These stories share a common thread: each woman approached intermittent fasting with a mindset of curiosity, patience, and self-compassion. Their successes didn't happen overnight, but through consistency and dedication, they achieved meaningful transformations.

Real testimonials like these remind us that intermittent fasting is not just a health tool, it's a path to rediscovering vitality and joy at any age. These women's journeys offer inspiration and encouragement for anyone considering taking the first step.

Results Achieved and Lessons Learned

The journeys of women over 60 who have embraced intermittent fasting reveal a wide range of transformative results, both physical and emotional. These stories demonstrate that fasting is not just about weight loss—it's about reclaiming energy, confidence, and control over one's health. Along the way, these women have also learned valuable lessons that can inspire and guide others.

Results Achieved

Many women report noticeable changes in their physical health, including:

- **Improved weight management**: Fasting has helped reduce stubborn fat, particularly around the midsection, a common challenge after menopause.
- **Enhanced energy levels**: Women often describe feeling more alert and energetic throughout the day, with fewer afternoon slumps.

- **Better blood sugar control**: For those managing conditions like type 2 diabetes, fasting has stabilized glucose levels and improved insulin sensitivity.
- **Reduced inflammation**: Many women note improvements in joint pain, digestion, and overall mobility, likely due to fasting's anti-inflammatory effects.
- **Improved sleep quality**: Better alignment with natural circadian rhythms has led to deeper, more restorative sleep.

Beyond physical changes, women also report emotional and mental benefits:

- **Greater confidence**: Achieving health goals through fasting has boosted self-esteem and reinforced a sense of empowerment.
- **Improved focus and clarity**: Fasting has helped women feel more mentally sharp and present in their daily lives.
- **Better relationship with food**: Many women say fasting has helped them move away from emotional eating and embrace mindful eating habits.

Lessons Learned

These transformations didn't happen overnight, and each woman's journey was marked by valuable insights and lessons:

1. **Consistency is Key:** Fasting works best when approached with a steady and realistic routine. Many women emphasize the importance of sticking to a schedule, even when life gets busy, and making adjustments when needed.
2. **Start Small and Build Confidence:** Jumping into long fasting periods can feel overwhelming. Starting with shorter fasting windows and

gradually extending them allowed these women to adapt without feeling deprived or stressed.

3. **Focus on Quality Nutrition:** Fasting is most effective when paired with a balanced diet. Prioritizing nutrient-dense foods during eating windows, such as lean proteins, healthy fats, and whole grains, maximized the benefits and kept energy levels stable.

4. **Listen to Your Body:** One of the most important lessons was learning to recognize and respond to their body's signals. Fasting is a flexible tool, and adapting it to suit energy levels, hunger patterns, and lifestyle needs is crucial for long-term success.

5. **Mindset Matters:** Approaching fasting with patience, curiosity, and self-compassion made the process more enjoyable. Many women found that focusing on progress rather than perfection helped them stay motivated and resilient.

6. **It's Never Too Late:** Perhaps the most inspiring lesson is that it's never too late to take charge of your health. Whether their goal was weight loss, increased energy, or better overall well-being, these women proved that age is no barrier to transformation.

A Journey of Empowerment

The results and lessons from these women's experiences highlight the incredible potential of intermittent fasting. By committing to the process, embracing flexibility, and focusing on overall wellness, they've achieved meaningful changes that extend far beyond the physical. Their journeys stand as proof that fasting is not just a method, it's a pathway to greater confidence, vitality, and fulfillment.

Common Mistakes to Avoid

What to Do When Fasting Doesn't Seem to Work

Intermittent fasting can be incredibly effective, but it's not uncommon to encounter periods when progress slows or results don't meet expectations. If fasting doesn't seem to be working for you, it's important to evaluate your approach, identify potential obstacles, and make adjustments. Here are some strategies to get back on track.

Reassess Your Fasting Method

Not all fasting methods work for everyone. If your current routine feels unsustainable or ineffective, consider experimenting with a different approach. For example:

- If the 16/8 method feels too restrictive, try starting with a 12/12 schedule to ease into fasting.
- If weight loss has plateaued, you might explore the 5:2 method or occasional 24-hour fasts to reset your metabolism.

Adapting your fasting style to suit your body and lifestyle can make a significant difference.

Evaluate Your Eating Window

Even with fasting, what you eat during your eating window is crucial. Overeating, consuming processed foods, or neglecting essential nutrients can hinder progress. To optimize your results:

- Focus on balanced meals that include lean proteins, healthy fats, and fiber-rich carbohydrates.

- Avoid sugary snacks, refined carbs, and overly processed foods that can disrupt blood sugar and energy levels.

Paying closer attention to the quality and portion size of your meals can reignite progress.

Hydration and Beverages

Sometimes, fasting appears ineffective because of hidden calorie intake. Beverages like coffee with cream, sugary teas, or flavored drinks can inadvertently break your fast. Stick to water, black coffee, or herbal teas during fasting periods, and ensure you're staying hydrated throughout the day.

Monitor Stress Levels

Chronic stress can interfere with the benefits of fasting by elevating cortisol levels, which promote fat storage and disrupt sleep. If stress is affecting your progress:

- Incorporate relaxation techniques such as meditation, yoga, or breathing exercises into your daily routine.
- Focus on sleep hygiene, aiming for 7–8 hours of restful sleep each night to support your body's recovery.

Reducing stress can improve your body's response to fasting and enhance overall well-being.

Check Your Activity Level

Fasting works best when paired with physical activity. If you've been sedentary, consider incorporating light exercise such as walking, yoga, or stretching. Gradually add strength training or cardio to support weight management and energy balance.

However, avoid overexertion, especially during fasting periods, as it can lead to fatigue and stress on the body. Find a routine that complements your energy levels and fasting schedule.

Give It Time

Fasting is not a quick fix; it's a long-term lifestyle change. Results may take weeks or months to become noticeable. If you've only recently started, be patient and focus on consistency. Monitor non-scale victories, such as improved energy, better sleep, or reduced cravings, which can be early signs of progress.

Seek Professional Guidance

If fasting still doesn't seem to work despite your best efforts, consider consulting a healthcare professional or nutritionist. They can help you identify any underlying health conditions, such as hormonal imbalances or thyroid issues, that may be affecting your progress.

Stay Flexible and Positive

Plateaus and challenges are normal in any lifestyle change. Approach these moments as opportunities to learn about your body and refine your routine. Staying flexible and maintaining a positive mindset ensures that intermittent fasting remains a sustainable and effective tool for your health journey.

By evaluating your habits, making small adjustments, and staying consistent, you can overcome obstacles and rediscover the benefits of intermittent fasting. Sometimes, a little patience and fine-tuning are all it takes to get back on track.

Chapter Seven

Solutions for Specific Situations

Fasting and Health Issues

Tips for Those with Diabetes, High Blood Pressure, or Arthritis

Intermittent fasting can be a powerful tool for improving health, even for those managing chronic conditions like diabetes, high blood pressure, or arthritis. However, it's essential to approach fasting with caution and tailor the practice to suit your specific health needs. Below are practical tips for safely incorporating fasting while managing these conditions.

Diabetes

For individuals with diabetes, particularly type 2 diabetes, fasting can improve insulin sensitivity and help stabilize blood sugar levels. However, it's crucial to proceed with medical guidance to avoid complications like hypoglycemia.

- **Work with Your Doctor**: Consult your healthcare provider before starting fasting, especially if you're taking medications such as insulin or glucose-lowering drugs, as dosages may need adjustment.
- **Start Gradually**: Begin with shorter fasting windows, such as 12/12, to observe how your body responds before transitioning to longer periods like 16/8.
- **Focus on Low-Glycemic Foods**: During eating windows, choose foods that have a low impact on blood sugar, such as leafy greens, whole grains, lean proteins, and healthy fats.
- **Monitor Blood Sugar Regularly**: Check your glucose levels before, during, and after fasting periods to ensure they remain stable.
- **Stay Hydrated**: Dehydration can exacerbate blood sugar fluctuations, so drink plenty of water throughout the day.

High Blood Pressure

Fasting can lower blood pressure by reducing weight, improving insulin sensitivity, and decreasing inflammation. To maximize these benefits safely:

- **Stay Hydrated**: Adequate hydration is essential for maintaining healthy blood pressure levels. Herbal teas and water are excellent choices during fasting periods.
- **Choose Potassium-Rich Foods**: During eating windows, focus on foods like bananas, avocados, and spinach, which support healthy blood pressure by balancing sodium levels.
- **Limit Sodium**: Avoid processed and salty foods, which can cause blood pressure spikes. Instead, season meals with herbs and spices.

- **Avoid Overexertion**: While light exercise like walking is beneficial, avoid intense workouts during fasting if they make you feel lightheaded or fatigued.
- **Monitor Your Blood Pressure**: Keep a record of your readings to identify any changes and discuss them with your doctor.

Arthritis

For those with arthritis, fasting can help reduce inflammation, which is a key driver of joint pain and stiffness. To support joint health and manage symptoms:

- **Incorporate Anti-Inflammatory Foods**: During eating periods, prioritize foods rich in omega-3 fatty acids (like salmon, walnuts, and flaxseeds) and antioxidants (such as berries, spinach, and turmeric).
- **Avoid Trigger Foods**: Limit processed foods, refined sugars, and trans fats, which can exacerbate inflammation.
- **Choose Gentle Exercises**: Low-impact activities like yoga, swimming, or tai chi can improve mobility and reduce joint discomfort. Avoid high-impact exercises that strain your joints.
- **Hydrate Regularly**: Adequate hydration can help lubricate joints and reduce inflammation.
- **Listen to Your Body**: If fasting increases fatigue or pain, consider shorter fasting windows or consult your doctor about modifications.

General Tips for Managing Chronic Conditions While Fasting

- **Start Slowly**: Ease into fasting with shorter durations to monitor how your body responds.
- **Focus on Balanced Nutrition**: Ensure your meals are nutrient-dense and include lean proteins, healthy fats, and complex carbohydrates.

- **Stay Flexible**: Adjust your fasting schedule if you feel unwell or if your condition requires more frequent meals.
- **Seek Professional Guidance**: Regular check-ups with your doctor or a nutritionist can ensure fasting is both safe and effective for your condition.

By approaching fasting thoughtfully and tailoring it to your health needs, you can harness its benefits while managing diabetes, high blood pressure, or arthritis. A balanced, informed strategy ensures that fasting becomes a valuable part of your overall wellness plan.

When to Consult a Doctor

Intermittent fasting can offer many health benefits, but it's essential to ensure that it's safe and appropriate for your specific situation, especially if you're managing existing health conditions or taking medications. Consulting a doctor before starting or modifying a fasting routine is a critical step in maintaining safety and achieving the best results.

Who Should Consult a Doctor Before Fasting

1. **Individuals with Chronic Conditions:** If you have diabetes, high blood pressure, arthritis, or any other chronic health condition, it's important to discuss fasting with your healthcare provider. They can help tailor a fasting plan to your needs, monitor your progress, and adjust medications if necessary.

2. **Those on Medications:** Certain medications, especially those for blood sugar, blood pressure, or heart conditions, may need adjustments when fasting. For example, skipping meals can affect how medications are absorbed or lead to low blood sugar levels.

3. **People with a History of Disordered Eating:** Fasting can trigger unhealthy behaviors in individuals with a history of eating disorders, such as binge eating or severe restriction. A healthcare professional can help assess whether fasting is a suitable choice.

4. **Women Experiencing Significant Fatigue or Dizziness:** Persistent fatigue, dizziness, or other symptoms while fasting could indicate an underlying issue or an imbalance in your fasting routine. Seeking medical advice ensures your safety.

5. **Individuals with Unexplained Symptoms:** If you experience symptoms like severe headaches, extreme hunger, or gastrointestinal discomfort that interfere with daily life, consulting a doctor can help identify the cause and determine if fasting is the right choice.

What to Discuss with Your Doctor

When consulting a doctor about intermittent fasting, be prepared to discuss:

- **Your health history**: Mention any chronic conditions, medications, or past challenges with dieting.
- **Your fasting goals**: Explain why you want to fast, whether for weight management, energy improvement, or overall health.
- **Your intended fasting method**: Share your plan, such as the 16/8 or 5:2 method, and ask if it's appropriate for your needs.
- **Any symptoms or concerns**: Mention any discomfort or issues you've experienced while fasting, such as dizziness, fatigue, or difficulty sleeping.

When to Stop Fasting and Seek Immediate Help

Stop fasting and consult a doctor immediately if you experience:

- Severe or persistent dizziness, fainting, or confusion.

- Extreme hunger that interferes with daily activities.
- Sudden changes in blood sugar levels, particularly if you have diabetes.
- Significant weight loss that seems unhealthy or unintentional.
- Intense physical or emotional distress related to fasting.

The Role of Professional Guidance

A healthcare professional or nutritionist can provide personalized advice, monitor your progress, and ensure that fasting is safe and effective. They can also suggest modifications to your fasting plan or recommend alternative strategies if fasting isn't suitable for your situation.

By consulting a doctor and seeking professional guidance, you can approach intermittent fasting with confidence and peace of mind, knowing that your health and safety are prioritized. This step not only helps prevent potential risks but also maximizes the benefits of fasting for your unique needs.

Travel and Social Life

How to Manage Fasting During Vacations or Social Occasions

Intermittent fasting doesn't have to be put on hold during vacations or social events. With a little planning and flexibility, you can maintain your fasting routine while enjoying special moments and staying true to your health goals. Here are practical strategies to help you balance fasting with travel and social activities.

Be Flexible with Your Schedule

While consistency is important, it's okay to adjust your fasting routine to fit your travel plans or social events. For example, if a dinner party extends past your usual eating window, allow yourself some flexibility and resume your regular schedule the following day. Occasional deviations won't derail your progress.

Choose Fasting-Friendly Methods

Certain fasting methods, such as the 12/12 or 16/8 schedule, are easier to adapt during travel or social occasions. These methods provide flexibility and allow you to align your eating window with group activities, such as shared meals or events.

Plan Ahead When Traveling

When traveling, a little preparation can help you stick to your fasting routine:

- Research your destination for healthy food options and restaurants that align with your eating goals.
- Pack travel-friendly snacks like nuts, seeds, or dried fruit for your eating window to avoid relying on processed foods.
- Time your meals around travel schedules, such as eating before a flight or after a long drive, to make fasting periods more convenient.

Focus on Balanced Choices at Social Events

Social gatherings often come with indulgent foods and drinks, which can feel challenging to navigate. During your eating window:

- Prioritize nutrient-dense options, such as salads, lean proteins, and whole grains, if available.
- Enjoy treats in moderation without guilt, remembering that fasting is about balance, not restriction.

- Stay hydrated with water or unsweetened beverages, especially if alcohol is served.

Communicate Your Needs

If you're comfortable, share your fasting routine with friends or family. Most people are understanding and supportive of health-related goals. This can make it easier to politely decline snacks outside your eating window or request meal times that align with your schedule.

Use Fasting-Free Days Strategically

Vacations or special occasions can be a great time to incorporate a more relaxed fasting method, such as the 5:2 approach. On non-fasting days, you can fully enjoy social meals while still maintaining the structure of your fasting lifestyle.

Listen to Your Body

Travel and social events can be physically and mentally demanding, so prioritize how you feel. If fasting becomes too stressful during these occasions, it's okay to pause and resume later. The most important thing is to enjoy the moment and return to your routine when ready.

Key Takeaway

Intermittent fasting is a flexible tool that can adapt to the rhythm of your life. By planning ahead, staying mindful of your choices, and allowing for flexibility, you can maintain your health goals without sacrificing the joy of travel and social connections. Remember, the goal is balance, fasting is a lifestyle, not a rigid rulebook.

Adjustments for a Flexible Lifestyle

Adapting Fasting for Challenging Days

Life isn't always predictable, and there will be days when sticking to your fasting routine feels particularly difficult. Whether it's due to stress, unexpected events, or a demanding schedule, intermittent fasting doesn't have to be an all-or-nothing approach. Adapting your routine for difficult days allows you to maintain progress while honoring your body's needs.

Listen to Your Body

Difficult days are often a signal that your body needs something different. If you're feeling unusually hungry, fatigued, or overwhelmed, it's okay to modify your fasting schedule. Shorten your fasting window or choose a more relaxed method, like the 12/12 approach, to give yourself some breathing room.

Focus on Nutrition Over Timing

When fasting feels challenging, prioritize the quality of your meals over strict adherence to your schedule. Eating nutrient-dense foods, such as lean proteins, healthy fats, and fiber-rich vegetables, helps stabilize energy levels and supports your overall well-being, even if your fasting window is shorter than usual.

Incorporate Mini-Fasts

On days when a full fasting schedule feels overwhelming, consider mini-fasts. For example, try fasting for 10–12 hours instead of 16, allowing yourself more flexibility without abandoning the practice entirely. This can help you maintain the habit while reducing stress.

Stay Hydrated

Fatigue or hunger during difficult days is often a sign of dehydration. Drinking plenty of water, herbal teas, or black coffee during fasting periods can help you feel more energized and reduce hunger pangs.

Adjust to Stressful Situations

Stress can make fasting harder, as elevated cortisol levels can trigger cravings and hunger. On particularly stressful days:

- Practice mindfulness or relaxation techniques, such as deep breathing or yoga, to manage stress without turning to food.
- Allow yourself a small, nutrient-rich snack, such as a handful of nuts or a boiled egg, to curb hunger and maintain focus.

Keep Moving

Gentle physical activity, like walking or stretching, can help boost energy and reduce feelings of restlessness on difficult days. Exercise also supports mental clarity, making it easier to stick to your adjusted fasting routine.

Embrace Flexibility

Remember, fasting is a tool to support your health, not a rigid set of rules. Adjusting your routine to accommodate life's challenges is a sign of strength, not failure. Allowing for flexibility ensures that fasting remains sustainable and enjoyable, even during difficult times.

Plan for Recovery

After a challenging day, ease back into your regular routine gradually. Use the experience as an opportunity to learn what works for your body and refine your approach. Whether it's adjusting your fasting schedule, focusing on specific nutrients, or incorporating stress management techniques, small changes can make a big difference.

By making thoughtful adjustments on difficult days, you can maintain your commitment to intermittent fasting without compromising your well-being. Flexibility is the key to a sustainable fasting lifestyle, one that supports you through both easy and challenging moments.

Chapter Eight

Simple Recipes to Support Fasting

Quick and Easy Meals

Recipes for Breakfast, Lunch, and Dinner

Planning simple, nutrient-dense meals during your eating window is essential for supporting your fasting lifestyle. Here are easy and quick recipes for breakfast, lunch, and dinner that prioritize balanced nutrition while being delicious and satisfying.

Breakfast Recipes

1. Greek Yogurt Parfait
- **Ingredients**:
  o 1 cup plain Greek yogurt
  o ½ cup mixed berries (blueberries, strawberries, raspberries)

- o 1 tablespoon chia seeds
- o 1 tablespoon chopped nuts (almonds or walnuts)
- o Drizzle of honey (optional)
- **Instructions**:
- o Layer Greek yogurt, berries, and chia seeds in a bowl or glass.
- o Top with chopped nuts and a light drizzle of honey for sweetness.
- o Enjoy immediately for a high-protein, antioxidant-rich start to your day.

2. Avocado Toast with Egg

- **Ingredients**:
- o 1 slice whole-grain bread
- o ½ avocado, mashed
- o 1 boiled, poached, or fried egg
- o Pinch of salt, pepper, and red pepper flakes (optional)
- **Instructions**:
- o Toast the bread and spread the mashed avocado on top.
- o Add the egg and season with salt, pepper, and red pepper flakes.
- o Serve with a side of fresh spinach or arugula.

Lunch Recipes

1. Grilled Chicken Salad

- **Ingredients**:
- o 2 cups mixed greens (spinach, arugula, or kale)
- o 1 grilled chicken breast, sliced
- o ½ avocado, sliced
- o ½ cup cherry tomatoes, halved
- o 2 tablespoons olive oil
- o 1 tablespoon lemon juice

- o Salt and pepper to taste
  - **Instructions**:
- o Arrange the greens, chicken, avocado, and cherry tomatoes in a bowl.
- o Whisk olive oil and lemon juice together, then drizzle over the salad.
- o Toss gently and season with salt and pepper.

2. Quinoa and Roasted Vegetable Bowl
  - **Ingredients**:
- o 1 cup cooked quinoa
- o 1 cup roasted vegetables (zucchini, sweet potatoes, bell peppers)
- o 1 tablespoon tahini or hummus
- o 1 teaspoon olive oil
- o Pinch of cumin or smoked paprika
  - **Instructions**:
- o Arrange the quinoa and roasted vegetables in a bowl.
- o Drizzle with tahini or hummus and olive oil.
- o Sprinkle with cumin or smoked paprika for added flavor.

Dinner Recipes

1. Baked Salmon with Steamed Vegetables
  - **Ingredients**:
- o 4 oz salmon fillet
- o 1 cup steamed broccoli and carrots
- o 1 teaspoon olive oil
- o 1 tablespoon lemon juice
- o Pinch of garlic powder, salt, and pepper
  - **Instructions**:
- o Preheat the oven to 375°F (190°C).

- Season the salmon with garlic powder, salt, and pepper, then drizzle with olive oil and lemon juice.
- Bake for 12–15 minutes or until cooked through.
- Serve with steamed broccoli and carrots on the side.

2. Turkey and Vegetable Stir-Fry

- **Ingredients**:
- 4 oz ground turkey
- 1 cup mixed stir-fry vegetables (snap peas, bell peppers, mushrooms)
- 1 teaspoon sesame oil
- 1 tablespoon low-sodium soy sauce
- 1 teaspoon grated ginger (optional)
- **Instructions**:
- Heat sesame oil in a skillet over medium heat.
- Cook the ground turkey until browned.
- Add vegetables and stir-fry until tender-crisp.
- Stir in soy sauce and ginger, then serve warm.

These quick and easy recipes provide the balanced nutrition you need to complement your fasting routine. Each dish is rich in essential nutrients, simple to prepare, and perfect for women looking to maintain energy and vitality while supporting their intermittent fasting journey.

Additional Easy and Quick Breakfast Recipes

1. Spinach and Feta Egg Muffins

- **Ingredients**:
- 4 large eggs
- 1 cup fresh spinach, chopped

- ¼ cup crumbled feta cheese
- Salt and pepper to taste

Instructions:
- Preheat oven to 350°F (175°C) and grease a muffin tin.
- Whisk the eggs in a bowl and stir in the spinach, feta, salt, and pepper.
- Pour the mixture evenly into muffin tin cups.
- Bake for 18–20 minutes or until set.
- Store leftovers in the fridge for a grab-and-go breakfast.

2. Banana Almond Butter Smoothie

Ingredients:
- 1 ripe banana
- 1 tablespoon almond butter
- 1 cup unsweetened almond milk
- 1 tablespoon chia seeds
- ½ teaspoon cinnamon

Instructions:
- Blend all ingredients until smooth.
- Pour into a glass and enjoy.
- Add a handful of ice cubes for a chilled smoothie or oats for a heartier texture.

3. Overnight Oats with Peanut Butter and Chocolate

Ingredients:
- ½ cup rolled oats
- 1 cup unsweetened almond milk
- 1 tablespoon natural peanut butter
- 1 teaspoon cocoa powder
- 1 teaspoon honey or maple syrup (optional)

- **Instructions**:

o Combine oats, almond milk, peanut butter, cocoa powder, and honey in a jar or container.

o Stir well, cover, and refrigerate overnight.

o In the morning, stir again and top with a few slices of banana or dark chocolate shavings for extra flavor.

4. Cottage Cheese and Fruit Bowl

- **Ingredients**:

o 1 cup low-fat cottage cheese

o ½ cup pineapple chunks or peach slices

o 1 tablespoon flaxseeds or chia seeds

o 1 teaspoon honey (optional)

- **Instructions**:

o Scoop the cottage cheese into a bowl.

o Top with pineapple or peach slices and sprinkle with flaxseeds.

o Drizzle honey on top for a touch of sweetness.

5. Sweet Potato Breakfast Hash

- **Ingredients**:

o 1 small sweet potato, peeled and diced

o 1 tablespoon olive oil

o ½ cup diced bell peppers

o 1 egg

o Salt, pepper, and paprika to taste

- **Instructions**:

o Heat olive oil in a skillet over medium heat.

o Add diced sweet potato and cook for 5–7 minutes until softened.

o Stir in bell peppers and cook for another 2–3 minutes.

o Push the vegetables to one side of the skillet and crack an egg into the empty space.

o Cook the egg to your preferred doneness and season with salt, pepper, and paprika.

o Serve as a hearty, nutrient-dense breakfast.

These quick breakfast recipes are designed to fuel your body with protein, fiber, and healthy fats, setting you up for success in your intermittent fasting routine. They are simple to prepare and perfect for busy mornings!

Additional Easy and Quick Lunch Recipes

1. Tuna and Avocado Salad

- **Ingredients**:

o 1 can of tuna in water, drained

o ½ avocado, mashed

o 1 cup mixed greens (spinach, arugula, or kale)

o 1 tablespoon olive oil

o Juice of ½ lemon

o Salt and pepper to taste

- **Instructions**:

o In a bowl, mix the tuna and mashed avocado until combined.

o Place the greens on a plate, top with the tuna mixture, and drizzle with olive oil and lemon juice.

o Season with salt and pepper, then toss gently before serving.

2. Caprese Wrap

- **Ingredients**:

o 1 whole-grain wrap

- 3 slices of fresh mozzarella
- 1 medium tomato, sliced
- Fresh basil leaves
- 1 teaspoon balsamic glaze
- Salt and pepper to taste

Instructions:
- Lay the wrap flat and layer the mozzarella, tomato slices, and basil leaves in the center.
- Drizzle with balsamic glaze and season with salt and pepper.
- Roll the wrap tightly and enjoy!

3. Chickpea and Cucumber Bowl

Ingredients:
- 1 cup canned chickpeas, rinsed and drained
- ½ cup diced cucumber
- ¼ cup diced red onion
- 1 tablespoon olive oil
- 1 teaspoon red wine vinegar
- 1 teaspoon dried oregano

Instructions:
- Combine the chickpeas, cucumber, and red onion in a bowl.
- Drizzle with olive oil and red wine vinegar, then sprinkle with oregano.
- Mix well and serve as a light, refreshing lunch.

4. Turkey and Hummus Roll-Ups

Ingredients:
- 4 slices of deli turkey
- 2 tablespoons hummus

- 4 cucumber sticks
- 4 carrot sticks

- **Instructions**:

- Spread a thin layer of hummus onto each slice of turkey.
- Place one cucumber stick and one carrot stick at one end of the slice, then roll it up tightly.
- Repeat for all slices and enjoy as a protein-packed lunch.

5. Mediterranean Quinoa Bowl

- **Ingredients**:

- 1 cup cooked quinoa
- ½ cup diced cucumber
- ½ cup cherry tomatoes, halved
- ¼ cup crumbled feta cheese
- 2 tablespoons kalamata olives, sliced
- 1 tablespoon olive oil
- Juice of ½ lemon

- **Instructions**:

- In a bowl, combine the quinoa, cucumber, cherry tomatoes, feta, and olives.
- Drizzle with olive oil and lemon juice, then toss to combine.
- Serve immediately or store in the fridge for a ready-to-go lunch.

These lunch recipes are quick to prepare, packed with nutrients, and ideal for fueling your body during your eating window. They're perfect for busy days while keeping you satisfied and energized!

Additional Easy and Quick Dinner Recipes

1. Baked Cod with Lemon and Garlic
- **Ingredients**:
  - 4 oz cod fillet
  - 1 teaspoon olive oil
  - Juice of ½ lemon
  - 1 garlic clove, minced
  - Salt, pepper, and parsley to taste
  - 1 cup steamed green beans or asparagus (side)
- **Instructions**:
  - Preheat the oven to 375°F (190°C).
  - Place the cod on a baking sheet lined with parchment paper.
  - Drizzle with olive oil and lemon juice, and sprinkle with garlic, salt, and pepper.
  - Bake for 12–15 minutes or until the fish flakes easily with a fork.
  - Serve with steamed green beans or asparagus on the side.

2. Turkey Lettuce Wraps
- **Ingredients**:
  - 4 oz ground turkey
  - 1 teaspoon sesame oil
  - 1 tablespoon low-sodium soy sauce
  - 1 teaspoon grated ginger (optional)
  - 4 large lettuce leaves (e.g., butter lettuce or romaine)
  - Diced cucumber or shredded carrots (optional topping)

Instructions:
- Heat sesame oil in a skillet over medium heat.
- Add ground turkey and cook until browned, breaking it up with a spoon.
- Stir in soy sauce and ginger, cooking for 1–2 more minutes.
- Spoon the turkey mixture into the lettuce leaves and top with cucumber or carrots.
- Fold and enjoy as a light, flavorful dinner.

3. Shrimp Stir-Fry with Vegetables

- **Ingredients:**
  - 4 oz shrimp, peeled and deveined
  - 1 cup mixed stir-fry vegetables (e.g., bell peppers, broccoli, snap peas)
  - 1 teaspoon coconut oil or sesame oil
  - 1 tablespoon low-sodium soy sauce
  - 1 teaspoon sesame seeds (optional)

- **Instructions:**
  - Heat the oil in a large skillet or wok over medium heat.
  - Add the shrimp and cook for 2–3 minutes until pink. Remove and set aside.
  - Add vegetables to the skillet and stir-fry until tender-crisp.
  - Return the shrimp to the skillet, drizzle with soy sauce, and toss to combine.
  - Sprinkle with sesame seeds if desired, then serve.

4. Zucchini Noodles with Pesto and Cherry Tomatoes

- **Ingredients:**
  - 2 medium zucchinis, spiralized into noodles
  - 2 tablespoons pesto (store-bought or homemade)

- ½ cup cherry tomatoes, halved
- 1 tablespoon olive oil
- Grated Parmesan (optional)

- **Instructions**:
- Heat olive oil in a skillet over medium heat.
- Add the zucchini noodles and sauté for 2–3 minutes until just softened.
- Stir in the pesto and cherry tomatoes, cooking for 1 more minute.
- Sprinkle with Parmesan if desired, then serve immediately.

5. Grilled Chicken with Sweet Potato Mash

- **Ingredients**:
- 4 oz grilled chicken breast
- 1 medium sweet potato, peeled and diced
- 1 teaspoon butter or olive oil
- Pinch of cinnamon and salt
- Steamed spinach or broccoli (optional side)

- **Instructions**:
- Boil the sweet potato in a pot of water until tender, about 10–12 minutes. Drain and mash with butter, cinnamon, and salt.
- Grill the chicken breast until fully cooked, about 6–8 minutes per side.
- Serve the chicken alongside the sweet potato mash and steamed spinach or broccoli for a hearty, balanced meal.

These dinner recipes are designed to be quick, simple, and packed with essential nutrients. They provide satisfying and flavorful options to keep you on track with your fasting goals while making dinnertime stress-free.

Healthy Snacks to Break Your Fast

Breaking your fast with nutrient-dense snacks is a great way to gently reintroduce food to your system and set the tone for your eating window. These healthy snacks are light, easy to prepare, and packed with essential nutrients to fuel your body.

1. Greek Yogurt with Berries
- **Ingredients**: ½ cup plain Greek yogurt, ¼ cup mixed berries (blueberries, raspberries, or strawberries).
- **Why It's Great**: Greek yogurt is rich in protein, while berries provide antioxidants and natural sweetness.

2. Avocado Toast
- **Ingredients**: 1 slice of whole-grain bread, ½ avocado mashed, sprinkle of salt and pepper.
- **Why It's Great**: This snack is packed with healthy fats and fiber, making it satisfying and easy to digest.

3. Hard-Boiled Eggs with Veggies
- **Ingredients**: 1–2 hard-boiled eggs, cucumber slices, and carrot sticks.
- **Why It's Great**: Eggs are a protein powerhouse, and the veggies add fiber and hydration.

4. Smoothie
- **Ingredients**: 1 small banana, 1 tablespoon almond butter, 1 cup unsweetened almond milk, 1 teaspoon chia seeds.
- **Why It's Great**: A smoothie is gentle on the stomach and provides a balanced mix of protein, healthy fats, and natural sugars.

5. Hummus with Veggie Sticks

- **Ingredients**: 2 tablespoons hummus, sliced bell peppers, celery sticks, or cucumber.
- **Why It's Great**: Hummus offers plant-based protein and healthy fats, while the veggies add crunch and hydration.

6. Cottage Cheese with Pineapple

- **Ingredients**: ½ cup low-fat cottage cheese, ¼ cup pineapple chunks.
- **Why It's Great**: Cottage cheese is high in protein and calcium, while pineapple provides a burst of natural sweetness and vitamin C.

7. Apple Slices with Almond Butter

- **Ingredients**: 1 small apple, 1 tablespoon almond or peanut butter.
- **Why It's Great**: The fiber in the apple and the healthy fats in the almond butter make this a satisfying and energizing snack.

8. Nuts and Seeds Mix

- **Ingredients**: A handful of almonds, walnuts, and sunflower seeds (about ¼ cup).
- **Why It's Great**: A quick, nutrient-dense snack loaded with healthy fats, protein, and minerals.

9. Rice Cake with Smoked Salmon

- **Ingredients**: 1 brown rice cake, 1–2 slices of smoked salmon, a squeeze of lemon.
- **Why It's Great**: A light and protein-packed snack that feels indulgent while being healthy.

10. Banana and Chia Pudding

- **Ingredients**: ½ cup almond milk, 2 tablespoons chia seeds, ½ banana sliced.

- **Why It's Great**: A great source of omega-3 fatty acids and fiber, this pudding is easy to prepare and gentle on the stomach.

Each of these snacks is designed to break your fast gently while providing the nutrients and energy your body needs to transition into your eating window. Choose the one that fits your taste and enjoy the benefits of a balanced, satisfying start to your day!

Drinks for Fasting

Herbal Teas, Broths, and Beneficial Infusions

During fasting periods, staying hydrated is essential to support your body's natural processes and curb hunger. Herbal teas, broths, and infusions can provide soothing, health-boosting benefits while keeping your fasting practice intact. Here are some options for each category to complement your fasting routine.

Herbal Teas

1. **Chamomile Tea**

o **Benefits**: Chamomile tea is calming and helps reduce stress, making it an excellent choice during evening fasting hours to promote relaxation and better sleep.

Preparation:
- Boil 1 cup of water.
- Add 1–2 teaspoons of dried chamomile flowers or a chamomile tea bag.
- Cover and let steep for 5–7 minutes.

- Strain (if using loose flowers) and enjoy warm, plain, or with a slice of lemon if desired.

2. **Peppermint Tea**

o **Benefits**: Known for its digestive properties, peppermint tea can help soothe bloating, reduce hunger pangs, and keep you refreshed during fasting periods.

Preparation:

- Boil 1 cup of water.
- Add 1–2 teaspoons of dried peppermint leaves or a peppermint tea bag.
- Steep for 5–10 minutes, depending on how strong you like the flavor.
- Strain (if using loose leaves) and serve hot or chilled.

3. **Ginger Tea**

o **Benefits**: Ginger tea is anti-inflammatory and supports digestion. It's a great option to ease nausea or enhance circulation, particularly during longer fasts.

Preparation:

- Peel and slice a 1-inch piece of fresh ginger.
- Boil 1 cup of water and add the ginger slices.
- Simmer for 10 minutes, then strain into a cup.
- For added flavor (post-fast), you can add a dash of lemon juice.

Broths

1. **Bone Broth**

o **Benefits**: While not calorie-free, bone broth is nutrient-dense and can be incorporated into modified fasting routines. It provides collagen, amino acids, and minerals that support joint and gut health.

Preparation:
- In a large pot, combine 2–3 lbs of bones (chicken, beef, or fish) with water to cover them.
- Add a splash of apple cider vinegar to help extract nutrients.
- Simmer for 12–24 hours on low heat, skimming off impurities occasionally.
- Strain the broth and store in jars. Warm up a cup to sip during modified fasting.

2. **Vegetable Broth**

o **Benefits**: A low-calorie option for those looking to break their fast gently. Vegetable broth delivers hydration and electrolytes with a light, savory flavor.

Preparation:
- In a pot, combine 2–3 cups of chopped vegetables (carrots, celery, onions, and zucchini) with 8 cups of water.
- Add herbs like thyme, parsley, and bay leaves.
- Simmer for 1–2 hours, then strain and store. Reheat as needed for a light, nutrient-rich drink.

3. **Miso Broth**

o **Benefits**: This fermented broth offers probiotics and umami flavor. It's perfect for a post-fast boost, providing a gentle transition to eating while supporting digestion.

- **Preparation**:

o Boil 2 cups of water.

o In a separate bowl, dissolve 1–2 tablespoons of miso paste in a small amount of warm water.

o Stir the dissolved miso into the hot water and mix until smooth.

o Add chopped scallions or seaweed for extra flavor (optional).

Infusions

1. **Lemon Water**

o **Benefits**: A simple infusion of water with fresh lemon slices helps cleanse the digestive system, provides vitamin C, and refreshes the palate. Drink it during fasting for added hydration and a mild flavor.

Preparation:

- Slice half a lemon into thin rounds.
- Add the slices to a pitcher of water (1–2 liters).
- Let sit for at least 30 minutes before drinking, or refrigerate overnight for a stronger infusion.

2. **Cucumber and Mint Water**

o **Benefits**: This refreshing infusion combines cucumber's hydrating properties with mint's cooling and digestive benefits. It's perfect for a light, spa-like drink during fasting.

Preparation:

- Thinly slice ½ cucumber and add it to a pitcher of water.
- Add 5–6 fresh mint leaves and stir.
- Let infuse for 1–2 hours in the refrigerator for a refreshing drink.

3. **Apple Cider Vinegar Infusion**

o **Benefits**: Apple cider vinegar aids digestion, stabilizes blood sugar, and reduces cravings. Consume it diluted, especially before breaking your fast, to ease digestion.

Preparation:

- Add 1–2 teaspoons of apple cider vinegar to a glass of cold or lukewarm water.
- Stir well.

- For added flavor (post-fast), you can mix in a pinch of cinnamon or a slice of lemon.

Tips for Preparation

- **Fresh Ingredients**: Use fresh herbs, vegetables, and spices whenever possible for the best flavor and nutrient content.
- **Batch Cooking**: Broths and infusions can be made in larger quantities and stored in the refrigerator for up to 4–5 days.
- **Serving Temperature**: Serve teas and broths warm for a soothing effect or chilled for a refreshing option, depending on your preference.

How to Incorporate These Drinks

- **During Fasting Periods**: Stick to calorie-free options like herbal teas and plain infused water to stay hydrated without breaking your fast.
- **Post-Fasting**: Light broths or apple cider vinegar infusions are ideal for easing into your eating window, preparing your digestive system for nutrient-dense meals.

These drinks not only support hydration but also enhance the health benefits of fasting, keeping you refreshed, focused, and energized throughout your routine.

The Importance of Hydration

Hydration plays a vital role in supporting your overall health and well-being, especially during intermittent fasting. Staying properly hydrated ensures that your body can function optimally, maintain energy levels, and handle the natural processes that occur during fasting periods. For women over 60, hydration is even more critical, as the body's ability to retain water naturally decreases with age.

Why Hydration Is Essential During Fasting

1. **Supports Metabolism:** Water is essential for metabolic processes, including the breakdown of fat for energy during fasting. Proper hydration helps your body efficiently utilize stored energy, making fasting more effective.

2. **Reduces Hunger and Cravings:** Often, feelings of hunger are actually signs of dehydration. Drinking water or herbal teas during fasting can suppress hunger and help you stay comfortable throughout your fasting period.

3. **Promotes Detoxification:** Fasting naturally encourages your body to detox by repairing cells and eliminating waste. Hydration supports this process by flushing out toxins and maintaining healthy kidney and liver function.

4. **Prevents Fatigue and Dizziness:** Dehydration can lead to symptoms like low energy, dizziness, or headaches—common issues during fasting. Drinking enough water ensures that your body stays energized and balanced.

5. **Improves Skin and Joint Health:** Hydration helps maintain skin elasticity and reduces dryness, both of which are important as you age. It also lubricates joints, reducing stiffness and discomfort, which can improve mobility.

How Much Water Do You Need?

While water needs vary by individual, a general guideline is to aim for at least 8–10 cups (64–80 ounces) of water per day. However, during fasting, you may need more to compensate for fluid lost through metabolism and normal bodily functions.

Listen to your body and adjust based on factors like activity level, climate, and how long your fasting window lasts.

Tips to Stay Hydrated During Fasting

- **Start Your Day with Water**: Begin your day with a glass of water to rehydrate after sleep and set the tone for hydration throughout the day.
- **Drink Regularly**: Sip water consistently during fasting hours rather than drinking large amounts all at once.
- **Incorporate Herbal Teas**: Herbal teas like chamomile, peppermint, or ginger provide hydration with added calming or digestive benefits.
- **Add Electrolytes**: If you're fasting for extended periods or exercising, consider adding a pinch of sea salt or electrolyte tablets to your water to replenish minerals.
- **Use Infused Water**: Add slices of cucumber, lemon, or mint to make water more appealing and refreshing.

Signs You May Need More Hydration

Be aware of the signs of dehydration so you can take action quickly. These include:

- Feeling thirsty or having a dry mouth.
- Dark yellow urine or infrequent urination.
- Fatigue or dizziness.
- Dry skin or lips.

If you notice these signs, increase your water intake immediately and monitor your symptoms.

Hydration Beyond Fasting Periods

Hydration doesn't stop when your fasting window ends. Continue drinking water during your eating periods to support digestion, nutrient absorption, and overall recovery. This practice complements the benefits of fasting and ensures your body remains balanced.

Hydration is a simple yet powerful tool for enhancing the benefits of intermittent fasting. By prioritizing your water intake and staying mindful of your body's needs, you can make your fasting experience more effective, enjoyable, and supportive of long-term health.

Chapter Nine

Frequently Asked Questions

Answers to the Most Common Concerns

Can I Fast If I Am Over 70 Years Old?

Yes, you can practice intermittent fasting after the age of 70, but it's important to approach it with care and consideration for your body's unique needs. At this stage of life, fasting can still provide significant health benefits, such as improved digestion, better blood sugar control, reduced inflammation, and even enhanced energy levels. However, it is essential to ensure that fasting is safe and appropriate for your specific circumstances.

Factors to Consider Before Fasting

1. **Your Overall Health:** Before starting intermittent fasting, consult with your healthcare provider, especially if you have chronic conditions

like diabetes, hypertension, or heart disease. These conditions don't necessarily prevent you from fasting, but adjustments to your fasting routine or medication schedule may be required.

2. **Nutritional Needs:** As you age, your body's nutritional needs change. You may require more protein to maintain muscle mass, more calcium and vitamin D for bone health, and sufficient fiber for digestion. Fasting should never compromise your ability to meet these needs. During your eating window, focus on nutrient-dense foods like lean proteins, healthy fats, whole grains, fruits, and vegetables.

3. **Energy Levels:** Energy fluctuations are common as you age, so it's important to choose a fasting method that aligns with your natural energy patterns. If you're new to fasting, start with a gentler approach, such as the 12/12 method, where you fast for 12 hours (including sleep) and eat within a 12-hour window. You can gradually extend the fasting period as your body adjusts.

4. **Medication and Fasting:** Many people over 70 take medications that may require food to avoid side effects. If this applies to you, consult your doctor to explore safe ways to incorporate fasting while managing your medication schedule.

Benefits of Fasting for People Over 70

1. **Improved Metabolic Health:** Intermittent fasting can help stabilize blood sugar levels and improve insulin sensitivity, which is particularly beneficial for older adults managing type 2 diabetes or prediabetes.

2. **Reduced Inflammation:** Chronic inflammation contributes to age-related conditions such as arthritis and heart disease. Fasting promotes cellular repair and reduces inflammation, potentially alleviating symptoms.

3. **Enhanced Digestion:** Fasting gives the digestive system a rest, reducing bloating and improving overall gut health.

4. **Promotes Longevity:** Studies suggest that fasting may stimulate processes like autophagy, which helps remove damaged cells and supports overall cellular health. This could contribute to healthy aging and increased vitality.

Tips for Safe Fasting After 70

- **Start Slowly**: Begin with shorter fasting windows and increase gradually as your body becomes accustomed to the practice.
- **Hydrate Consistently**: Proper hydration is crucial during fasting, as dehydration can lead to dizziness or fatigue. Drink water, herbal teas, or infused water throughout the day.
- **Focus on Nutrient-Dense Meals**: Use your eating window to prioritize balanced meals with sufficient calories and nutrients. Avoid processed or sugary foods that provide empty calories.
- **Listen to Your Body**: Pay attention to how you feel during fasting periods. If you experience persistent fatigue, dizziness, or other symptoms, adjust your fasting schedule or consult a healthcare provider.
- **Be Flexible**: Life can be unpredictable, so allow yourself the flexibility to modify your fasting routine on days when your energy levels are lower or during special occasions.

When to Avoid Fasting

There are certain situations where fasting may not be advisable, especially if:

- You are underweight or have experienced significant weight loss.
- You have a history of eating disorders.

- You experience severe fatigue, dizziness, or other symptoms during fasting.
- Your doctor advises against fasting due to specific medical conditions or treatments.

Intermittent fasting can be a powerful tool for improving health and well-being at any age, including after 70. By taking a thoughtful and personalized approach, you can enjoy the benefits of fasting safely and sustainably. Always prioritize your body's needs and consult a healthcare professional to ensure that fasting is right for you.

Does Fasting Cause Muscle Loss?

A common concern about intermittent fasting is whether it leads to muscle loss. While muscle loss can occur during extended periods of severe calorie restriction or malnutrition, intermittent fasting, when done properly, does not typically result in muscle loss. In fact, it can help preserve and even promote muscle health when combined with adequate nutrition and physical activity. Let's explore this in more detail.

Understanding Muscle Loss and Fasting

Muscle loss occurs when the body breaks down muscle protein to use as energy, typically when it lacks sufficient calories or nutrients from food. However, intermittent fasting is not a starvation diet—it's a controlled eating pattern that cycles between periods of fasting and eating. When practiced correctly, it encourages the body to burn stored fat for energy while preserving lean muscle mass.

Why Fasting Does Not Typically Cause Muscle Loss

1. **Hormonal Adaptations During Fasting**

o **Human Growth Hormone (HGH)**: Fasting stimulates the production of HGH, a hormone that plays a key role in muscle maintenance, fat metabolism, and cellular repair. Elevated HGH levels help protect muscle tissue, especially during fasting periods.

o **Insulin Sensitivity**: Fasting improves insulin sensitivity, which enhances the body's ability to use nutrients efficiently during the eating window, reducing the need to break down muscle for energy.

2. **Body's Preference for Fat Burning:** During fasting, the body primarily relies on fat stores for energy, not muscle protein. This shift to fat-burning (ketosis) ensures that muscle tissue is preserved while the body uses stored fat as its primary fuel source.

3. **Short Duration of Fasting Periods:** Intermittent fasting typically involves shorter fasting windows (e.g., 16 hours), which are not long enough to trigger significant muscle breakdown. Extended fasts lasting several days are more likely to result in muscle loss, but these are not part of standard intermittent fasting practices.

How to Prevent Muscle Loss While Fasting

1. **Adequate Protein Intake:** Consuming enough protein during your eating window is crucial for preserving muscle mass. Aim for 20–30 grams of protein per meal, depending on your body weight and activity level. Great protein sources include lean meats, fish, eggs, dairy, legumes, and plant-based options like tofu or quinoa.

2. **Incorporate Strength Training:** Regular resistance training or weight-bearing exercises stimulate muscle growth and prevent muscle

breakdown. Fasting does not impair your ability to build or maintain muscle when combined with strength training.

3. **Consume Nutrient-Dense Meals:** Focus on balanced meals that include proteins, healthy fats, and complex carbohydrates. These nutrients provide the energy and building blocks your body needs to preserve muscle while fasting.

4. **Stay Hydrated:** Dehydration can lead to muscle cramps and fatigue, so ensure you're drinking plenty of water throughout the day. Proper hydration supports muscle function and overall performance.

5. **Break Your Fast Wisely:** Start your eating window with a meal that includes protein and healthy carbohydrates to replenish energy stores and support muscle recovery. For example, a grilled chicken salad with quinoa or a smoothie made with Greek yogurt and berries can be an excellent choice.

What the Research Says

Studies show that intermittent fasting is not associated with significant muscle loss when paired with proper nutrition and exercise. For instance, research comparing intermittent fasting to traditional calorie-restricted diets found that individuals practicing intermittent fasting maintained similar or better muscle mass while losing fat.

When Muscle Loss May Occur

While intermittent fasting is generally safe for muscle preservation, muscle loss can happen if:

- **Protein intake is insufficient**: Failing to meet your daily protein needs can lead to muscle breakdown over time.
- **Calorie intake is too low**: Prolonged calorie deficits, especially when combined with fasting, can result in muscle loss.

- **You're sedentary**: Without regular physical activity, especially resistance training, muscles can weaken and shrink regardless of diet or fasting.

Key Takeaway

Intermittent fasting, when done correctly, does not cause muscle loss. In fact, it can enhance fat burning while preserving lean muscle, thanks to hormonal adaptations and the body's ability to prioritize fat as an energy source. To protect your muscles, ensure you consume enough protein, engage in regular strength training, and focus on balanced nutrition during your eating windows. As always, listen to your body and consult a healthcare professional if you have concerns about your fasting routine.

Debunking Fasting Myths

Addressing Misconceptions About Fasting

Intermittent fasting is a popular health practice, but it's often surrounded by myths and misconceptions that can discourage people or lead to unnecessary fears. Let's break down some of the most common myths about fasting and reveal the truth behind them.

Myth 1: Fasting Slows Down Your Metabolism

The Truth: Contrary to popular belief, intermittent fasting does not slow your metabolism. In fact, short-term fasting can boost your metabolism by increasing levels of norepinephrine, a hormone that helps burn fat. Studies have shown that fasting for up to 48 hours may slightly increase metabolic rate. Long-term, excessive calorie restriction (not fasting) is what slows metabolism.

Myth 2: Fasting Causes Muscle Loss

The Truth: As discussed earlier, intermittent fasting does not lead to muscle loss when practiced correctly. Hormonal changes during fasting, such as increased human growth hormone (HGH), help preserve muscle mass. Pairing fasting with adequate protein intake and regular strength training ensures your muscles stay strong and healthy.

Myth 3: You'll Feel Tired and Weak All the Time

The Truth: While it's true that some people experience fatigue during the initial adjustment period, most find that their energy levels stabilize and even improve once their body adapts. Fasting promotes the use of stored fat for energy, which provides a steady, sustained source of fuel. Staying hydrated and eating nutrient-dense meals during your eating window also helps maintain energy levels.

Myth 4: Fasting Is Dangerous for Women Over 60

The Truth: Fasting can be safely practiced by women over 60 when approached thoughtfully. As long as you focus on nutrient-rich meals, stay hydrated, and listen to your body, fasting can be a healthy and sustainable lifestyle choice. Consulting with a healthcare provider ensures that fasting is tailored to your specific health needs.

Myth 5: Fasting Means Starving Yourself

The Truth: Fasting is not about starvation—it's a structured approach to eating that involves alternating periods of fasting and nourishment. Unlike starvation, intermittent fasting ensures you meet your nutritional needs during your eating window while giving your body time to rest and repair during fasting periods.

Myth 6: You Can't Exercise While Fasting

The Truth: Many people successfully combine fasting with exercise. Light to moderate activities like walking, yoga, or strength training are excellent during fasting periods. For higher-intensity workouts, you can time them during or after your eating window for optimal performance.

Myth 7: Fasting Is Just a Trend

The Truth: Fasting has been practiced for centuries across cultures and religions as a tool for health and spiritual well-being. Modern research confirms its scientific benefits, such as improved insulin sensitivity, reduced inflammation, and better metabolic health. Intermittent fasting is far from a passing trend—it's rooted in both tradition and science.

Myth 8: Fasting Is Only About Weight Loss

The Truth: While fasting can help with weight management, its benefits go far beyond the scale. Fasting promotes cellular repair, improves digestion, stabilizes blood sugar, and even supports brain health. Many people adopt fasting for its holistic health benefits rather than just weight loss.

Myth 9: You'll Be Hungry All the Time

The Truth: Hunger is common when first starting fasting, but it diminishes as your body adjusts. During fasting periods, your body learns to use stored fat as fuel, which helps reduce hunger over time. Drinking water or herbal teas can also help curb hunger pangs.

Myth 10: Fasting Is One-Size-Fits-All

The Truth: Fasting is highly customizable, with various methods (16/8, 5:2, alternate-day fasting) to suit individual needs. What works for one person may not work for another, and it's important to find a fasting routine that fits your lifestyle and health goals.

Key Takeaway

Myths about fasting can create unnecessary doubts and confusion, but understanding the science behind fasting clears up these misconceptions. Intermittent fasting is a safe, flexible, and evidence-based practice that offers numerous health benefits when approached with care and proper knowledge. By debunking these myths, you can approach fasting with confidence and make informed decisions about your health.

Chapter Ten

Maintaining Results Over Time

Turning Fasting Into a Habit

How to Avoid Regaining Weight

One of the most common concerns with any lifestyle change, including intermittent fasting, is the risk of regaining weight over time. While intermittent fasting can be an effective tool for weight loss, maintaining those results requires a sustainable approach. Here are strategies to help you avoid regaining weight and make fasting a lasting, successful habit.

1. Focus on Sustainable Fasting Methods

Choose a fasting schedule that fits your lifestyle and feels natural. Overly restrictive or complicated routines can lead to burnout, making it harder to stick with the practice long term. Sustainable methods like the 16/8 or 5:2 approach are easier to maintain and adapt as life changes.

2. Prioritize Nutrient-Dense Meals

What you eat during your eating window is just as important as when you eat. Focus on meals rich in lean proteins, healthy fats, whole grains, and plenty of vegetables. These nutrient-dense foods keep you full, stabilize blood sugar, and provide the energy you need to stay active. Avoid processed and high-sugar foods that can lead to overeating or energy crashes.

3. Practice Portion Control

Even with a structured fasting schedule, overeating during your eating window can lead to weight regain. Be mindful of portion sizes and eat until you're satisfied, not overly full. Listening to your body's hunger and fullness cues can help you strike the right balance.

4. Stay Consistent with Physical Activity

Regular exercise not only supports weight maintenance but also improves overall health and well-being. Combine strength training to preserve muscle mass with cardio or low-impact activities like walking or yoga to support fat burning and cardiovascular health. Aim to find activities you enjoy to make exercise a consistent part of your routine.

5. Manage Stress

Stress can lead to emotional eating and disrupt your fasting routine. Incorporate stress management techniques like mindfulness, meditation, or deep breathing exercises to maintain a sense of calm and control. Adequate sleep also plays a key role in reducing stress and preventing overeating.

6. Avoid an "All-or-Nothing" Mindset

Life can be unpredictable, and it's normal to deviate from your fasting routine occasionally. Don't let one indulgent day or skipped fast derail your progress. Instead, focus on getting back on track with your next meal or fasting period. Consistency over time is more important than perfection.

7. Stay Hydrated

Proper hydration is essential for controlling appetite and preventing overeating. Drinking water, herbal teas, or other fasting-friendly beverages throughout the day can help reduce hunger pangs and keep your energy levels stable.

8. Track Your Progress

Keeping a journal or using an app to log your fasting schedule, meals, and activity can help you identify patterns and stay accountable. Regularly reflecting on your progress can keep you motivated and highlight areas for improvement.

9. Avoid Relying Solely on Fasting for Weight Maintenance

Intermittent fasting is a tool, not a magic solution. Combine it with other healthy habits like balanced nutrition, physical activity, and mindfulness to create a holistic approach to long-term health and weight management.

10. Celebrate Non-Scale Victories

Weight is just one measure of success. Pay attention to other benefits of fasting, such as improved energy, better digestion, and enhanced mental clarity. Celebrating these wins can help you stay motivated and focused on the bigger picture of your health journey.

Key Takeaway

Maintaining weight loss with intermittent fasting requires a thoughtful, balanced approach. By focusing on sustainable habits, mindful eating, regular activity, and stress management, you can turn fasting into a lasting lifestyle that supports your long-term health goals. Consistency and self-compassion are your greatest allies on this journey.

Creating a Maintenance Plan

A well-structured maintenance plan is essential for preserving the results achieved through intermittent fasting. It helps you stay consistent, balance your lifestyle, and prevent setbacks. Here's how to create a sustainable maintenance plan that fits your goals and routine.

1. Evaluate Your Current Routine

Start by assessing what has worked for you during your fasting journey. Consider the following:

- Which fasting method felt most manageable (e.g., 16/8, 5:2)?
- What eating patterns and meal choices helped you stay on track?
- Were there specific challenges or obstacles you overcame?

Understanding your successes and pain points allows you to design a plan that feels natural and achievable.

2. Choose a Sustainable Fasting Schedule

For maintenance, it's important to adopt a fasting schedule that complements your daily life. Some options include:

- **Flexible 16/8**: Continue fasting for 16 hours a day but allow occasional adjustments for social events or special occasions.

- **Modified 5:2**: Fast two non-consecutive days per week but relax the calorie restriction slightly for long-term adherence.
- **12/12 Schedule**: A gentler approach where you fast for 12 hours overnight and eat within a 12-hour window, ideal for periods when life feels busier.

3. Prioritize Balanced Nutrition

Maintaining results isn't just about when you eat but also what you eat. Ensure your meals are nutrient-dense and satisfying:

- **Protein**: Incorporate lean meats, fish, eggs, legumes, and plant-based proteins to support muscle maintenance and satiety.
- **Healthy Fats**: Include avocados, nuts, seeds, olive oil, and fatty fish for long-lasting energy and overall health.
- **Fiber**: Focus on whole grains, vegetables, and fruits to support digestion and stabilize blood sugar.
- **Hydration**: Stay hydrated with water, herbal teas, or infused waters to curb cravings and maintain energy.

Avoid excessive reliance on processed or sugary foods, which can disrupt your progress.

4. Incorporate Regular Exercise

Physical activity is a key part of a maintenance plan. Aim to:

- **Stay Active Daily**: Walk, stretch, or engage in light activities to keep your body moving.
- **Strength Train Weekly**: Build or maintain muscle mass with resistance exercises 2–3 times per week.
- **Include Cardio**: Support cardiovascular health with moderate aerobic exercise, such as swimming, cycling, or brisk walking.

Find activities you enjoy to make exercise a consistent and enjoyable part of your lifestyle.

5. Create a Weekly Meal Plan

Planning your meals in advance can reduce stress and help you stick to healthy habits.

- **Plan for Variety**: Rotate recipes and ingredients to avoid boredom.
- **Prep Ahead**: Batch cook or prepare ingredients like grains, vegetables, and proteins to make meal prep quicker.
- **Include Snacks**: Choose healthy snacks like nuts, yogurt, or hummus with veggies to prevent overeating during your eating window.

6. Allow for Flexibility

Life is unpredictable, and occasional deviations from your plan are normal. The key is to avoid guilt and return to your routine afterward. Flexibility keeps fasting sustainable and prevents burnout.

7. Monitor Your Progress

Track your progress to stay motivated and identify areas for improvement. You can:

- **Track Weight and Measurements**: Regularly monitor changes to ensure you're maintaining your goals.
- **Journal Your Habits**: Note how you feel, what works, and what challenges arise.
- **Celebrate Milestones**: Recognize and reward your commitment to maintaining your health.

8. Adjust As Needed

Your maintenance plan may need tweaks as your lifestyle evolves. For example:

- Shorten or lengthen fasting windows based on energy needs.

- Modify meal plans during vacations or social events.
- Adapt exercise routines to match your physical capabilities or preferences.

The ability to adapt your plan ensures it remains relevant and effective.

9. Set Long-Term Goals

Having long-term health goals provides direction and motivation. Your goals might include:

- Maintaining a stable weight.
- Improving fitness levels.
- Supporting overall wellness, such as better sleep, digestion, or energy.

Revisiting and refining your goals helps keep you focused and engaged.

Key Takeaway

A maintenance plan is a roadmap for sustaining the progress you've made with intermittent fasting. By combining a flexible fasting schedule, balanced nutrition, regular activity, and ongoing self-reflection, you can ensure lasting results and a healthier lifestyle. Remember, consistency and adaptability are the foundations of long-term success.

Monitoring Progress

Regular Check-Ups and Adjustments to the Plan

Monitoring your progress is an essential part of maintaining long-term success with intermittent fasting. Regular check-ups and making thoughtful adjustments to your plan allow you to stay aligned with your health goals and address any changes in your body's needs. This proactive approach ensures that fasting remains effective and sustainable over time.

The Importance of Regular Check-Ups

1. **Tracking Health Metrics**

Regular health check-ups provide valuable insights into your overall well-being. Key metrics to monitor include:

- Weight and body measurements.
- Blood sugar levels.
- Blood pressure and cholesterol.
- Bone density and muscle mass (especially important for women over 60).

These measurements help you identify trends and determine whether your fasting routine is supporting your health goals.

2. **Evaluating How You Feel**

Pay attention to how you feel physically, mentally, and emotionally. Questions to ask yourself include:

- Do you feel energized and alert?
- Are you sleeping well?
- Have you noticed improvements in digestion or mood?
- Are you experiencing any discomfort or fatigue?

Your overall sense of well-being is a crucial indicator of whether your plan is working or needs adjustment.

3. **Consulting Your Doctor or Nutritionist**

Regular consultations with a healthcare professional ensure your fasting plan is aligned with your health status. This is especially important if you have chronic conditions like diabetes or hypertension. A doctor or nutritionist can help you interpret health metrics, fine-tune your plan, and address any concerns.

Adjusting Your Plan

Intermittent fasting is not a static routine—it should evolve with your body and lifestyle. Regularly assessing your progress allows you to make informed adjustments to optimize results.

1. **Reassess Your Fasting Schedule**

Over time, your fasting needs may change. For example:

o If you feel too hungry or fatigued, shorten your fasting window (e.g., from 16/8 to 14/10).

o If you've plateaued with weight loss, try extending your fasting window slightly or incorporating a new method like the 5:2 approach.

2. **Adjust Nutrition Based on Goals**

As your body adapts, you may need to refine your dietary choices:

o **For energy levels**: Incorporate more complex carbohydrates and healthy fats.

o **For muscle maintenance**: Increase your protein intake, particularly if you're engaging in strength training.

o **For overall health**: Add more antioxidant-rich fruits and vegetables to support aging gracefully.

3. **Adapt to Lifestyle Changes**

Life events like travel, social commitments, or changes in work schedules may require temporary or permanent adjustments to your fasting routine. Flexibility is key to staying consistent without feeling overwhelmed.

4. **Address Plateaus or Challenges**

If progress slows, reassess your habits:

o Are you consuming too many or too few calories during your eating window?

o Are you staying hydrated and exercising regularly?

o Are stress or sleep issues interfering with your progress?

Small changes, like tweaking meal timing or prioritizing sleep, can help overcome challenges.

Tips for Long-Term Monitoring

- **Keep a Journal**: Record your fasting schedule, meals, energy levels, and emotions to identify patterns and areas for improvement.
- **Use Apps or Tools**: Digital tools can track fasting hours, calories, and health metrics, making monitoring more convenient.
- **Set Milestones**: Celebrate progress by setting small, achievable goals, such as improved energy or hitting a target weight.

The Value of Reflection

Take time every few months to reflect on your journey:
- Are you meeting your goals?
- What aspects of fasting feel effortless, and where do you struggle?
- How has your body and mindset changed since you started?

This reflection not only reinforces your commitment but also highlights areas where you can improve or adapt your plan.

Key Takeaway

Regular check-ups and adjustments ensure that intermittent fasting remains effective and aligned with your goals. By tracking your progress, consulting professionals, and staying flexible, you can sustain your health journey and enjoy the long-term benefits of fasting. Remember, the key to success is consistency, awareness, and adaptability.

A Future of Wellness

How Fasting Will Help You Live a Longer and Healthier Life

Intermittent fasting is more than a short-term health practice—it's a lifestyle that can promote longevity and enhance your quality of life. By incorporating fasting into your routine, you support your body's natural processes, reduce the risk of chronic diseases, and foster physical and mental well-being. For women over 60, fasting offers a sustainable path to aging gracefully while feeling strong, vibrant, and in control of your health.

1. Supports Cellular Repair and Longevity

Fasting activates a process called autophagy, where the body cleans out damaged cells and regenerates new ones. This "cellular recycling" improves overall health at the cellular level, reducing the risk of age-related diseases such as Alzheimer's, cancer, and cardiovascular conditions. By supporting this natural process, fasting helps slow down the aging process and promotes a longer, healthier life.

2. Improves Metabolic Health

As you age, the risk of metabolic disorders like diabetes and obesity increases. Intermittent fasting helps:

- Regulate blood sugar levels.
- Improve insulin sensitivity.
- Reduce visceral fat (fat around the organs). These benefits not only enhance your energy and overall health but also decrease the likelihood of developing chronic conditions that can shorten your lifespan.

3. Reduces Chronic Inflammation

Chronic inflammation is a significant contributor to age-related diseases, including arthritis, heart disease, and even certain cancers. Fasting lowers inflammatory markers in the body, promoting better joint health, improved mobility, and a reduced risk of inflammatory diseases.

4. Enhances Brain Health

Fasting doesn't just benefit your body—it also protects your brain. By reducing oxidative stress and inflammation, fasting promotes brain health and may lower the risk of cognitive decline. It also stimulates the production of brain-derived neurotrophic factor (BDNF), a protein that supports memory, learning, and overall cognitive function. This means you can stay sharper and more focused as you age.

5. Encourages Heart Health

Heart disease remains one of the leading causes of death worldwide, but fasting can help reduce this risk. Intermittent fasting:

- Lowers blood pressure.
- Reduces levels of LDL ("bad") cholesterol and triglycerides.
- Improves overall cardiovascular function. By prioritizing heart health, fasting supports longevity and helps you maintain an active, independent lifestyle.

6. Fosters a Balanced Lifestyle

One of the often-overlooked benefits of fasting is the structure and mindfulness it brings to your day. Fasting encourages you to be more intentional about what and when you eat, which can lead to healthier habits overall. This balance extends to other areas of life, such as sleep, stress management, and physical activity, all of which contribute to a longer, healthier life.

7. Boosts Energy and Vitality

Rather than draining you, fasting helps your body use energy more efficiently. By transitioning to fat as a primary fuel source, you may experience more stable energy levels throughout the day. This vitality allows you to stay active, pursue hobbies, and enjoy life to the fullest as you age.

8. Provides a Sense of Control and Empowerment

Intermittent fasting offers a simple yet powerful way to take charge of your health. By practicing fasting, you create a routine that supports both your physical and mental well-being, fostering a sense of empowerment. This mindset can positively impact your outlook on aging, helping you embrace the future with confidence and optimism.

A Healthier, Longer Life Awaits

Intermittent fasting is more than a tool for weight management or disease prevention, it's a practice that supports holistic wellness and longevity. By giving your body the space to heal, repair, and function optimally, fasting helps you age with strength, vitality, and grace.

The benefits of fasting go beyond the physical. It nurtures your mental clarity, emotional resilience, and sense of purpose, ensuring that the years ahead are filled with health, happiness, and fulfillment. With fasting as part of your routine, you're investing in a future where you can enjoy life to its fullest potential, every single day.

Conclusion

Celebrating Yourself

Final Reflections on Your Journey

As you reach the conclusion of this journey into intermittent fasting, take a moment to celebrate yourself, not just for the results you've achieved, but for the commitment, effort, and self-care you've embraced along the way. Adopting a lifestyle like intermittent fasting is not just about health or weight loss; it's a testament to your dedication to living a vibrant, empowered life.

Reflecting on Your Accomplishments

Pause and reflect on how far you've come since you started. Think about the challenges you've overcome, the habits you've changed, and the lessons you've learned. Whether it's feeling more energized, sleeping better, or gaining confidence in your ability to prioritize your health, every step forward is worth celebrating.

Each small victory, choosing a balanced meal, sticking to a fasting schedule, or simply listening to your body, is part of a larger transformation. These accomplishments are evidence of your resilience and determination.

Embracing the Long-Term Benefits

Your journey is about more than the physical changes you may have noticed. It's also about the long-term benefits you're investing in:

- A healthier, more energized body.
- A sharper, more focused mind.
- A renewed sense of confidence and self-worth.

These benefits extend far beyond the fasting periods and eating windows, they are tools for living a life of vitality, joy, and balance.

Acknowledging Your Growth

Intermittent fasting isn't always easy, and there may have been times when you doubted yourself or faced setbacks. But every step of this process has helped you grow, not just in health but in self-awareness and strength. By taking control of your habits and embracing change, you've proven that it's never too late to improve your well-being.

Looking Ahead with Confidence

The journey doesn't end here. Instead, you've laid the foundation for a lifestyle that will continue to evolve with you. As you move forward, remember that flexibility and balance are key. Celebrate your successes, learn from your challenges, and always prioritize your well-being.

By reflecting on what you've achieved and looking forward with optimism, you're not just maintaining a lifestyle, you're building a future full of health, energy, and confidence. This is your time to thrive, and you've earned every moment of it.

Celebrate yourself for embarking on this journey and for the courage and persistence it took to create lasting change. You've taken a powerful step toward living a life filled with vitality, and that is truly something to be proud of.

Motivation to Keep Going

Staying motivated is essential for maintaining the habits and lifestyle you've worked so hard to build. Motivation doesn't come from perfection, but from consistency, self-compassion, and the ability to recognize the deeper reasons behind your efforts. By focusing on the positive changes you've experienced and keeping your goals in mind, you can continue to thrive on your intermittent fasting journey.

Celebrate Your Wins

Acknowledge the progress you've made, both big and small. Whether it's weight management, improved energy levels, or simply feeling more in control of your health, every achievement matters. Reflecting on these wins reminds you of the positive impact fasting has had on your life and inspires you to keep going.

Connect with Your "Why"

Think back to why you started intermittent fasting in the first place. Was it to improve your health, regain energy, or feel more confident? Reconnecting with your original motivation can help you refocus and stay committed, especially on days when it feels more challenging.

Set New Goals

Having something to work toward can reignite your excitement. Your goals don't have to be weight-related. They might include trying new healthy recipes, increasing your strength through exercise, or improving your sleep habits. New goals keep the journey fresh and engaging.

Find Support

Surround yourself with people who support and encourage your efforts. This could include friends, family, or even online communities of like-minded individuals practicing intermittent fasting. Sharing experiences, tips, and successes can boost your motivation and remind you that you're not alone.

Focus on How You Feel

Pay attention to the physical and emotional benefits you've gained from fasting. Improved digestion, mental clarity, and better sleep are powerful motivators to maintain the lifestyle you've built. Use these positive changes as a reminder of why fasting works for you.

Reward Yourself

Set milestones for yourself and celebrate when you reach them. Rewards can be anything that makes you feel good, like treating yourself to a relaxing day, buying a new book, or trying a fun activity. Rewards reinforce your progress and make the journey enjoyable.

Be Flexible

Life is unpredictable, and there will be times when your fasting routine may need to be adjusted. Embrace flexibility as a strength, not a weakness. Allow yourself to make changes without guilt, and focus on returning to your routine when possible. This mindset keeps you motivated without unnecessary pressure.

Visualize Your Future Self

Imagine the person you're becoming by continuing with intermittent fasting, a healthier, more confident, and energized version of yourself.

Visualizing your future self can provide a powerful mental boost and help you stay on track.

Remember It's a Lifestyle

Fasting is not a quick fix; it's a sustainable way of living. By treating it as a long-term commitment to your health, you shift your focus from temporary results to lifelong well-being. This perspective fosters motivation that lasts.

Motivation is about progress, not perfection. By celebrating your journey, staying connected to your goals, and embracing the lifestyle you've created, you can continue to enjoy the benefits of fasting for years to come. Trust in your ability to stay consistent and know that every step forward is a step toward a healthier, happier you.

Call to Action

Encouragement to Share the Book and Personal Experiences

Your journey with intermittent fasting is unique, and your experience has the power to inspire others. Sharing what you've learned and how fasting has positively impacted your life can not only help others discover the benefits but also strengthen your own commitment to maintaining a healthy lifestyle.

Spread the Word

If you've found value in this book and in your own fasting practice, consider sharing it with those who could benefit. Whether it's a friend, family member, or colleague, sharing your experience might be the catalyst someone else needs to begin their own journey toward better health. By sharing the book, you help others access the knowledge and support they need to succeed.

Share Your Story

Your personal story is a powerful tool for encouraging others. Sharing how fasting has impacted your energy, health, or mindset can be motivating for those who may be unsure or hesitant. Whether you choose to share your journey on social media, in conversation, or through personal blogs or forums, your words could be the inspiration someone needs to take the first step.

Join a Community

There are many online communities and support groups focused on intermittent fasting. By participating in these communities, you can exchange tips, offer encouragement, and hear from others about their experiences. Whether through social media or specialized forums, connecting with like-minded individuals will keep you engaged and motivated while allowing you to help others.

Offer Guidance

If you have experience with fasting and feel confident in your knowledge, consider helping those who are just starting. Offering advice on how to begin, what to expect, and how to stay motivated can be incredibly valuable for others. Your guidance can make a significant difference in someone else's fasting journey.

Celebrate Together

Fasting is not just a personal journey, it's a shared experience. Celebrate your wins, milestones, and successes with others. Whether it's with friends, family, or an online community, celebrating together reinforces the power of community support and strengthens everyone's commitment to better health.

By sharing this book and your personal experiences, you are not just helping others improve their lives, you're creating a ripple effect of positive change. The more you share, the more you inspire, and the more you stay motivated in your own journey. Let your story be a part of the larger conversation about health, wellness, and the transformative power of intermittent fasting.

Appendices

1. 30-Day Fasting Plan

Detailed and Adaptable Schedule

This 30-day intermittent fasting plan is designed to help you gradually incorporate fasting into your lifestyle while allowing flexibility to suit your individual needs. The plan provides a step-by-step approach, starting with shorter fasting windows and progressively increasing them as your body adapts. Whether you're new to fasting or looking to refine your routine, this adaptable plan offers a clear roadmap for success.

Week 1: Easing Into Fasting (12/12 Schedule)

For the first week, focus on a 12-hour fasting window and a 12-hour eating window. This method is gentle and allows your body to adjust without feeling overwhelmed.

- **Fasting Window**: 8:00 PM to 8:00 AM
- **Eating Window**: 8:00 AM to 8:00 PM

Tips for Week 1:

- Avoid late-night snacking to maintain the fasting period.

- Focus on balanced meals with plenty of protein, healthy fats, and fiber during the eating window.
- Stay hydrated by drinking water, herbal teas, or black coffee during the fasting period.

Week 2: Transition to the 14/10 Schedule

In the second week, extend your fasting window to 14 hours and reduce the eating window to 10 hours. This shift encourages your body to begin relying more on stored energy.

- **Fasting Window**: 8:00 PM to 10:00 AM
- **Eating Window**: 10:00 AM to 8:00 PM

Tips for Week 2:

- Break your fast with a nutrient-dense meal, such as Greek yogurt with berries or avocado toast with eggs.
- Adjust meal times to ensure you feel satisfied within the 10-hour eating window.
- Listen to your body and modify the schedule slightly if needed.

Week 3: Progress to the 16/8 Schedule

By week three, aim for the classic 16-hour fasting window and an 8-hour eating window. This is one of the most popular and effective intermittent fasting methods.

- **Fasting Window**: 8:00 PM to 12:00 PM
- **Eating Window**: 12:00 PM to 8:00 PM

Tips for Week 3:

- Use the morning hours to focus on hydration and light activities like walking or yoga.
- Plan two to three balanced meals during the eating window.

- Include plenty of vegetables, lean proteins, and whole grains for sustained energy.

Week 4: Maintain or Explore Other Methods

In the final week, maintain the 16/8 schedule or experiment with other fasting methods, such as the 5:2 plan or alternate-day fasting, based on your preferences and goals.

5:2 Plan Example:
- Eat normally for five days of the week.
- Choose two non-consecutive days to restrict calorie intake (around 500–600 calories).

Alternate-Day Fasting Example:
- Fast for 24 hours every other day, consuming only calorie-free beverages during the fasting period.

Tips for Week 4:
- Choose a method that feels sustainable and aligns with your lifestyle.
- Reflect on your progress and how fasting has improved your energy, focus, or overall well-being.
- Be flexible and make adjustments as needed to ensure long-term success.

Adapting the Plan to Your Needs

This 30-day plan is a guideline and can be adjusted based on your schedule, energy levels, and goals. If you find a particular fasting window challenging, take a step back and revisit a shorter fasting period before progressing. Consistency and self-compassion are key to making fasting a lasting part of your routine.

By following this structured and adaptable plan, you'll give your body time to adjust to fasting while building confidence in your ability to sustain this healthy lifestyle. Use this plan as a starting point for creating long-term habits that support your health and well-being.

3. Glossary of Terms

Explanations of Scientific Terms Used in the Book

This glossary provides clear and concise definitions of the scientific and technical terms referenced throughout the book. Use it as a quick reference to deepen your understanding of intermittent fasting and its effects on your body.

Autophagy

The body's natural process of cleaning out damaged cells and recycling them to produce new, healthier cells. Triggered during fasting, autophagy promotes cellular repair and may reduce the risk of age-related diseases.

Ketosis

A metabolic state in which the body burns fat for fuel instead of carbohydrates. Ketosis typically occurs during fasting or low-carb diets and is associated with weight loss and increased energy levels.

Insulin Sensitivity

The body's ability to respond effectively to insulin, a hormone that regulates blood sugar levels. Improved insulin sensitivity means the body uses glucose more efficiently, reducing the risk of type 2 diabetes.

Inflammation

The immune system's response to injury, infection, or chronic stress. While acute inflammation is necessary for healing, chronic inflammation can contribute to diseases such as arthritis, heart disease, and diabetes. Fasting may reduce chronic inflammation.

Metabolic Flexibility

The body's ability to switch between burning carbohydrates and fats for energy. Improved metabolic flexibility is a key benefit of intermittent fasting, helping the body adapt to different energy sources.

Circadian Rhythm

The natural 24-hour cycle that regulates various biological processes, including sleep, metabolism, and digestion. Fasting aligned with your circadian rhythm (e.g., eating earlier in the day) may enhance the benefits of fasting.

Human Growth Hormone (HGH)

A hormone produced by the pituitary gland that promotes cell regeneration, muscle growth, and fat metabolism. Fasting boosts HGH levels, supporting muscle maintenance and fat loss.

Ghrelin

Often called the "hunger hormone," ghrelin signals the brain when it's time to eat. During fasting, ghrelin levels may rise temporarily but stabilize over time, helping control appetite.

Leptin

A hormone that signals the brain when the body has enough stored energy (fat) and doesn't need to eat. Improved leptin sensitivity through fasting can help regulate hunger and prevent overeating.

Visceral Fat

Fat stored around the abdominal organs, which is more harmful than subcutaneous fat. High levels of visceral fat are linked to an increased risk of chronic diseases, and fasting helps reduce visceral fat effectively.

Calorie Restriction

Reducing calorie intake without malnutrition. While calorie restriction is a traditional method of weight loss, intermittent fasting offers similar benefits without requiring constant monitoring of calories.

Oxidative Stress

An imbalance between free radicals and antioxidants in the body, leading to cell damage. Fasting helps reduce oxidative stress, supporting overall health and longevity.

Electrolytes

Minerals like sodium, potassium, and magnesium that are essential for hydration and muscle function. Maintaining electrolyte balance during fasting helps prevent fatigue and muscle cramps.

Fasting Window

The period during which you abstain from eating. This window varies depending on the fasting method (e.g., 16 hours in the 16/8 method).

Eating Window

The period during which you consume your meals, following the fasting period. A typical eating window might last 8 hours in the 16/8 fasting method.

Fat Adaptation

The process by which the body becomes efficient at burning fat for fuel instead of carbohydrates. Fat adaptation typically occurs after consistent fasting or a low-carb diet.

Hyperglycemia

A condition characterized by high blood sugar levels. Fasting can help prevent hyperglycemia by improving blood sugar control.

Hypoglycemia

Low blood sugar levels, which can cause dizziness, fatigue, or irritability. Proper meal planning and hydration help prevent hypoglycemia during fasting.

5:2 Method

A fasting method in which you eat normally for five days of the week and restrict calorie intake (around 500–600 calories) on two non-consecutive days.

16/8 Method

A popular fasting method where you fast for 16 hours and eat during an 8-hour window. This method is beginner-friendly and easy to incorporate into daily life.

This glossary is designed to clarify the key terms used throughout the book, empowering you to fully understand the science and practices behind intermittent fasting.

Bonus Chapter: Your Exclusive Fasting Tools

To make your intermittent fasting journey even easier and more effective, I've created two exclusive downloadable resources for you! These printable tools will help you stay organized, track your progress, and plan your meals effortlessly.

Intermittent Fasting Planner (100 Printable Pages): a customizable journal to track your fasting hours, meals, energy levels, and progress. Perfect for staying accountable and seeing real results over time.

Weekly Intermittent Fasting Menu (Full-Color Printable): a beautifully designed weekly meal planner and checklist to help you organize your fasting schedule and meals at a glance. Includes space for meal prep notes and reminders to keep you on track. These tools are designed to support your success, making fasting simple and structured. **Scan the QR code now and start using them today!**

Acknowledgments

As this book comes to a close, I want to take a moment to express my heartfelt gratitude to everyone who has been a part of its creation and to those who will take the time to read it. This book is not just a guide; it's a reflection of countless efforts, support, and inspiration from people who believe in the power of health and transformation.

To my family and friends, thank you for your unwavering encouragement and understanding during the countless hours spent researching and writing. Your love and support have been my foundation and my motivation.

To the researchers, scientists, and health professionals whose work has inspired much of the content in this book, I am deeply grateful for your dedication to understanding and advancing the fields of nutrition, fasting, and wellness. Your insights have provided the tools and knowledge that have made this guide possible.

To the readers, thank you for choosing this book as part of your health journey. Whether you are just beginning or are well on your way, your commitment to improving your life through intermittent fasting is an inspiration. It is my hope that this book serves as a helpful resource and empowers you to take control of your health with confidence and joy.

Finally, to those who shared their personal fasting experiences and success stories, your courage and honesty have added depth and meaning to these pages. Your journeys remind us all that transformation is possible at any stage of life.

This book is dedicated to you, the women who inspire, empower, and prove that health and vitality are ageless. Thank you for allowing me to be a small part of your journey.

With gratitude and hope,

Amanda Wells

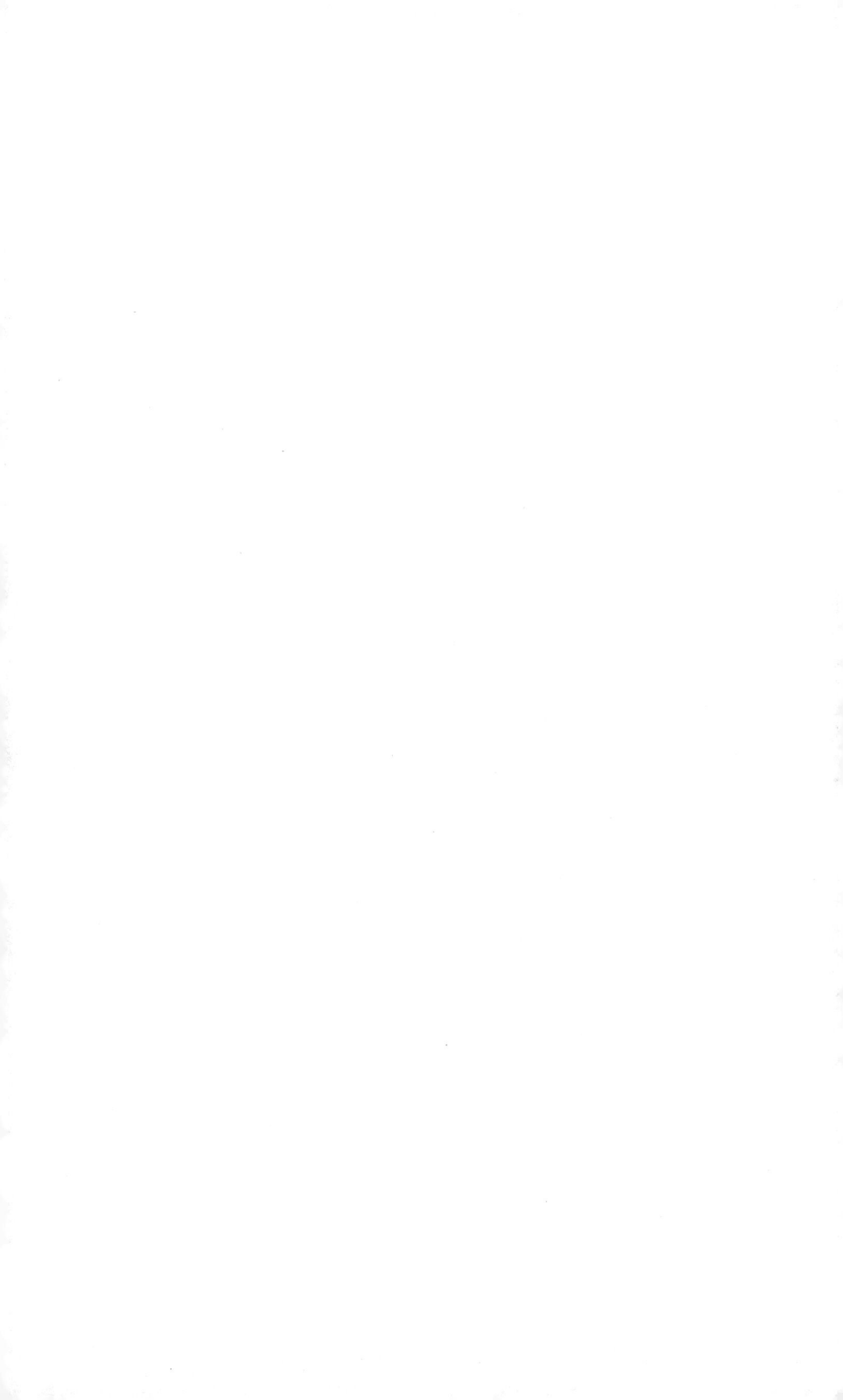

Made in United States
Cleveland, OH
03 June 2025